The 14-Day
Aromabeauty
Plan

How to look better, feel better

in 2 aromatic weeks

Maggie Tisserand

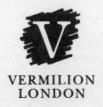

VERMILION
LONDON

This book is dedicated to the beauty that lies within.

First published in 1994

3 5 7 9 10 8 6 4 2

Copyright © Maggie Tisserand 1994

The moral right of Maggie Tisserand has been asserted in accordance with
the Copyright, Designs and Patents Act, 1988.

First published in the United Kingdom in 1994 by Vermilion
an imprint of Ebury Press
Random House, 20 Vauxhall Bridge Road, London SW1V 2SA

Random House Australia (Pty) Limited
20 Alfred Street, Milsons Point, Sydney, New South Wales 2061, Australia

Random House New Zealand Limited
18 Poland Road, Glenfield, Auckland 10, New Zealand

Random House South Africa (Pty) Limited
PO Box 337, Bergvlei, South Africa

Random House Canada
1265 Aerowood Drive, Mississauga, Ontario L4W 1B9, Canada

Random House UK Limited Reg. No 954009

A CIP catalogue record for this book is available
from the British Library.

ISBN 0 09 178247 3

Edited by Gillian Haslam
Designed by Clive Dorman
Typeset by Clive Dorman & Co.
Printed by Cox & Wyman Ltd., Reading, Berkshire

Contents

Introduction

We can all be likened to flowers in a garden, each with our own special colour, shape and size. But beyond that, we are fragrant flowers and our fragrance is our spirit. Just as the fragrance of the flower enhances its beauty, so our inner spirit, when allowed to shine through, enhances our beauty.

Every woman has her own concepts of beauty; this book reflects mine. To me, real beauty merges inner beauty, which we can call spirit or love, with outer beauty, which is our physical body. The most beautiful woman that I know has been blessed with an attractive physical appearance, but above and beyond this she radiates love, joy and contentment.

This is the ideal. In reality, most of us struggle with envy, and self-criticism. We compare ourselves (often unfavourably) to fashionable dictates of what constitutes beauty – supermodels, movie stars and princesses. But do we walk through a garden and judge the flowers? Do the flowers compare themselves to one another? Does the tulip want to be a rose? Why do we women constantly compare ourselves to illusions of beauty?

I will never be a willowy 5'8" supermodel or a voluptuous blonde bombshell, and to spend my life searching for this illusory perfection would be like chasing mirages in a desert: both a total waste of time and potentially very destructive. For me the answer lies in a mixture of realism – accepting the basic framework of my body – and optimism – the conviction that I can improve myself and become more beautiful, inside and out.

Just as I believe in holistic medicine to treat the whole person and not just the symptoms of illness, so I believe in the concept of holistic beauty care to beautify the *whole* woman, not just the outer layer of skin. This book presents a holistic beauty care plan based on my experience of using essential oils over the last 20 years, and though I am still a 5'4" freckled mother of three, I am sometimes mistaken for my daughter's sister and I haven't been seriously ill for years.

Not 'just another beauty book', *The 14-Day Aromabeauty Plan* is devised to help women increase the attractiveness of the body as well as to enhance inner health and vitality. Nor is this meant to be a medical book, though it is exciting to understand the workings of the human body. Hopefully you will find the *14-Day Aromabeauty Plan* an eminently versatile, practical, empowering and pleasurable way to improve the way you look and feel.

Anyone can use this plan, from teenagers to matriarchs and everyone in between. Whatever your lifestyle – whether a homemaker or a career woman, whether you believe in alternative medicine or not, whether you are financially comfortable or struggling on a budget – this plan is designed for you.

I hope this book will empower and encourage you to take responsibility for yourself rather than allowing the accrual of beauty problems which may one day require treatment by an outside expert. While not denying the benefits of visiting an aromatherapist, I do wish to expand the use of essential oils to women who for reasons of geography, finance or shyness have not yet experienced the rewards of aromatherapy. This aromabeauty plan does take dedication and concerted effort, but hopefully you'll also have a very enjoyable and enriching two weeks, indulging yourself in the beautiful and uplifting essential oils of nature, whilst becoming the most beautiful flower you can be.

Maggie Tisserand

Chapter 1

What is aromabeauty?

Aromabeauty is a term I coined to convey the use of aromatic or essential oils as an integral part of everyday beauty care. Essential oils for this purpose have, in my opinion, been insufficiently valued, and aromatherapy has generally been equated with putting right an illness either at home or by consulting an aromatherapist. However, this has not always been the case. In the ancient civilizations of Egypt, Greece and Rome, aromatics were used extensively, not only as medicines, but also as perfumes, skin unguents, massage oils and hair tonics, all designed to enhance overall beauty, sensuality and well-being. I feel it is now time to stop limiting the use of these precious essential oils to those moments when we are unwell, but to embrace them in everyday life so that we stay well, feel well and look well.

What are essential oils?

Within every aromatic plant or tree, there is a fragrant liquid which is the essence of the plant. This essence is both the fragrance of the flower and home to all the characteristics and properties of the plant. When the essence is separated from the flower through distillation, the resultant liquid is the essential oil. These oils are extremely complex and can be composed of hundreds of chemical constituents which imbue the plant with its distinctive aroma and particular qualities.

Essential oils are powerful substances and only very small

amounts are used at one time – for example, 6 to 10 drops in a full bath. Due to their concentration, it is crucial always to dilute the essential oils in a good quality fatty oil before applying them to the skin. While essential oils are extremely safe and non-toxic, some people with very sensitive skin cannot tolerate any fragranced product, including essential oils. Additionally, in a small number of people the citrus oils may cause irritation; if you suspect you may be one of these, it's wise to test a small area of skin first.

How do essential oils work on the body?

Essential oils are both applied to the skin and inhaled through the respiratory tract. Because they are composed of extremely tiny molecules, essential oils are able to penetrate the skin and enter the body. In this way an essential oil applied to the exterior travels within the lymphatic and circulatory systems to virtually every cell of the body. For example, by treating cellulite on the thigh with a blend of essential oils, we not only rid ourselves of the toxins causing the problem, but also stimulate the vital organs to work more efficiently and to bring about optimum metabolism. Essential oils also enhance the protective power of the immune system. In addition, essential oils are entirely natural and completely compatible with the body's own oils and fats, unlike commercial beauty preparations. Many of even the most expensive cosmetic creams contain lanolin, collagen, placenta extract and other animal products. Apart from whatever ethical objections you may have to using animal extracts, these commercial beauty aids derived from animals are unable to penetrate the skin, due to their large molecular size, and are therefore often ineffective. Unlike cosmetics that promise illusion in a jar, nature's essential oils deliver tangible results.

When inhaled, essential oil vapours enter the lungs to

circulate eventually within the bloodstream, or travel via the olfactory system to the brain where they affect our moods and emotions. Through their ability to permeate the skin and enter the body, the oils work in many ways to help regulate and heal. They may regenerate and strengthen cellular tissue. They replenish and repair skin cells and regulate the production of sebum. They cleanse and disinfect the skin, and help detoxify and remove poisons from the body. They strengthen the immune system, enabling us to fight disease, and they release stress and alleviate tension.

How do essential oils work in harmony with the lymphatic system?

The body's lymphatic system is a vitally important component in the maintenance of good health. Lymph permeates all the body tissues, removing toxins and bringing infection-fighting lymphocytes to wherever they are needed. Before toxins are excreted from the body, they must firstly pass through the lymph nodes where they are broken down and are then fed into the bloodstream, from where they then pass to the organs of elimination, and so make their way out of the body. When essential oils enter the body through the skin, either by massage, masks, bathing or any other method, they mix with lymph and are carried along on the same journey as the toxins. During this journey, the antiseptic, antiviral, antibiotic or anti-fungal properties of essential oils are able to kill off harmful organisms even before they reach the lymph nodes. Because there is less infective material passing into the lymph nodes, they rarely become inflamed and are better equipped to carry out their second function, which is to produce lymphocytes. The lymph also carries away excess fluids and fats from body tissues and organs – a function which prevents us from becoming obese and water-logged. Because essential oils perform an important role in keeping infection under control, the lymphatic system is able to carry off fats and fluids more easily, which means that our body shape, as well as our health, improves.

The lymphatic system is a part of the circulatory system and as such, is influenced by the heart . But the body systems are all interconnected, and according to the laws of acupuncture it is the lungs that govern the waterways of the body. The waterways refer to the lymphatic system, which means that as long as we are breathing, lymph is circulating around our body. It also means that any form of exercise that increases the action of the lungs is beneficial to the lymphatic system. Physical movement of the skin, such as skin brushing or massage, is also very beneficial to the free-flow of lymph.

What can essential oils do for you?

The effect of essential oils on the skin is profound. All essential oils are cleansing and antiseptic and certain essential oils, such as vetivert, encourage the skin to hold water and retain moisture. Others such as lavender promote the new growth of cells and help to rejuvenate the skin. Some oils, such as lemon, orange and bergamot, assist the body in carrying away toxins which improves skin clarity and tone. Whatever the problem, there is an aromatic solution.

This applies on many different levels, not only the skin and our visible selves, but also to our unseen psyche that can suffer and become over-burdened with stress. As we all know, stress is ageing, and on a bad day we can easily look ten years older than we are. The soothing and uplifting powers of essential oils help us let go of tension, and become more relaxed and peaceful.

To top it all off, essential oils are fun to use. Like a genie in a bottle waiting to emerge, the magic of essential oils is at your fingertips waiting for you to enjoy.

Is the 14-day aromabeauty plan for everyone?

This plan is for women of any age who wish to make a dramatic improvement in their bodies in a relatively short period of time. Whether you're a teenager or a granny, this book offers aromatherapy solutions to your particular problem area. There are, however, a few exceptions: this programme should *not* be used by pregnant or lactating women, or women who are under medical care. This is not to imply that essential oils are dangerous, but that the intensity of the programme and the resultant release of toxins would be inadvisable for women in these conditions.

Is it really possible to effect a change in 14 days?

Miracles don't happen overnight and long-standing problems require long-term effort. Ten years of neglect cannot be righted in a couple of weeks. However, by using this plan it is possible to start the process of regeneration and to attain tangible and pleasing results, but your commitment is crucial.

The power of essential oils, your determination to change, and your dedication of time and effort to this process are a potent combination. Success depends on all of these factors working together. By taking responsibility for yourself and by using the recommended blends of essential oils, you really can look better and feel better in only two aromatic weeks.

Chapter 2

The 14-Day Aromabeauty Plan

The 14-day aromabeauty plan is divided into two parts: everyday beauty care, which is really basic maintenance, and specific problem areas to be worked on, such as cellulite in the thighs, wrinkly knees or a sallow complexion.

There's also a third component which involves all the common sense requirements for vibrant health: restful sleep, a well-balanced diet, plenty of water, and exercise (I enjoy long walks in the woods near my home).

Without all three it is not possible to attain truly glowing good looks. If we smoke twenty cigarettes a day, eat junk food and survive on coffee and biscuits, no amount of beauty care can compensate the body for our neglect and abuse.

Everyday aromabeauty

Everyday we wash, we clean our teeth, we perform various rituals that are basic to hygiene and comfort. By using essential oils on a daily basis we can add an 'essential' bonus to our skin and our body.

I recommend a daily aromatic bath with any of numerous fragrant oils. Some of my favourite bath oils are lavender, especially at night since it is very soothing, geranium, myrtle or bergamot. An aromatic bath not only cleanses the skin, but also works on a deeper level to heal us and enhance our overall sense of well-being.

Cleansing and moisturizing the face with essential oils is vitally important in our often polluted environment. Filthy city streets, centrally heated houses, air-conditioned offices all affect our face, which is always naked and exposed to the world. We also need to feed and nourish the skin of the face everyday, just as we nourish our bodies with the food we eat. Essential oils are nature's 'skin foods'; they repair and revitalize our skin cells, allowing us to look our radiant best.

Another everyday area is our hands – always in and out of water, unprotected from the elements, or in contact with chemicals such as shampoo or washing-up liquid. Many of us neglect our hands, regarding them as tools and not as an integral part of the body beautiful. Daytime barrier and night-time protective hand creams help to keep out unwanted influences from our environment, replacing lost natural oils and water, as well as softening and rejuvenating our hard-working hands.

Problem spots

This book is divided into ten body areas with a chapter devoted to each. Each chapter concentrates on typical problems relevant to that body area, for example:

The face Dry and dehydrated skin; greasy skin; maturing skin; double chin; after-effects of spots; tired and irritated eyes; crow's feet; thin eyelashes; dry and chapped lips.

Hair and head Dry lack-lustre hair; dandruff; excess grease; hair loss; tension in head; stressed-out feeling.

Breasts Sagging breasts; breasts too large or too small; stretch marks; blemishes.

Back and shoulders Congested, blemished skin; greasy skin; dull-looking skin; tension in neck and shoulders.

Tummy and waist Excess fat; wrinkles; stored tension in solar plexus.

Thighs and buttocks Cellulite; obesity; stretch marks; buttock 'droop'; dull and lifeless skin.

Upper arms, neck and elbows Flabby upper arms; cellulite; excess fat; wrinkled elbows; neck lines; rough elbows; dry skin.

Knees, ankles and feet Fat knees; puffy knees; wrinkly knees; puffy ankles; hidden ankles; tired feet.

Hands and nails Dry skin; dehydrated skin; fat or puffy hands; brittle nails; ridged nails.

The plan

Appraisal

Before deciding which area to work on, evaluate yourself. Stand naked in front of a long mirror, not when you are feeling irritable and stressful, but after a relaxing bath would be a good time. Take an objective look – not a harsh critical judgement bemoaning the overindulgence in chocolates and cakes which have generated the lumps and bulges – but a kindly look merely to see where improvement could take place. Do the thighs feel a little tender to the touch and are they dimpled with cellulite? Are the knees a little fat or wrinkled? Have the round contours of the buttocks merged into the tops of the thighs? Is the upper chest spotty? Does the skin of the upper arms sag a little when you lift your arms? And what of the face? Is the skin as taut as you would like it to be and is the appearance of the skin smooth and clear?

Try to categorize your problem spots according to their importance to you. My lifestyle is fairly sedentary as I spend a lot of time writing books like this, and my upper thighs and buttocks really suffer. I periodically need to spend some time conscientiously working on them with my essential oil blends, so that they meet with my approval. Do the same for yourself: be honest but realistic. Take into account your age, your bone structure, your genetics, your lifestyle. If you're large and big boned, don't imagine that massage with essential oils will make you petite.

Looking in the mirror, use the following chart to record those problem areas you consider to be major, moderate or minor and make a note of your initial evaluation of yourself, as it is very hard to remember at the end of fourteen days what you looked like at the beginning. It's also important to see how far you've progressed in a relatively short time, to give yourself confidence and the commitment to continue working towards your goal.

Aromabeauty Evaluation Chart

Date:

Body Problem	Major	Moderate	Minor

Allocating Time

Whether you are working in an office or taking care of children at home, you will need to set some time aside for you and your beauty plan, as the time could easily be swallowed up by your everyday routine.

How much time you devote is up to you, but once decided, try to commit to it every day for at least 14 days. I work on a 14-day beauty plan 365 days a year, concentrating on different parts of the body; hopefully your first 14 days will just be the beginning of a lifetime of aromabeauty.

I recommend a minimum of one hour a day in order to see an improvement. Of course, if you have more time or if you want to make an all out effort before a special occasion like a wedding or a holiday, spend as much time as you wish (bearing in mind the need for patience, as discussed in Chapter 4). For most of us, time is precious and it's fortunate that many of the beauty regimes recommended in this book can be done while you're relaxing in front of the television or listening to music.

Don't try to cram too much into one 14-day period. Quality is more important than quantity. You've got the rest of your life – just make a start.

If it is a problem to find the time to spend on yourself, then I recommend that you focus on those areas which are of major concern to you, making a note of body problems which you consider to be moderate or minor so that you can address these whenever you can find the time. For example, if you find that having just given up smoking after many years you have a lifeless sallow skin, which you want to repair, this is a major problem and requires a lot of attention in order to achieve tangible results in a two-week period. Be realistic about the time you can devote to yourself, and follow the 14-day chart for sallow skin, with commitment and dedication. Select a moderate problem such as wrinkly knees, and perhaps one or two minor problems such as dry lips and lack-lustre hair to include in your 14-day beauty plan, should there be a suitable opportunity.

If, however, you have decided that you have two major problems that require urgent care like droopy buttocks and cellulite on the thighs, and you know that one hour is the absolute maximum you will be able to spend on yourself each day, then it's best not to attempt much more. Just follow the 14-day chart for thighs and buttocks.

Refer back to the Aromabeauty Evaluation Chart and carefully select your major, moderate and minor problem areas for this 14-day period. The blank chart below will help you develop your own personalized beauty regimen.

If you wish to improve your body generally and increase vitality rather than concentrate on a specific body area, follow the 14-day aromabeauty blitz in chapter 15, which will take between 1 hour 10 minutes and 1 hour 30 minutes, each day. This is on top of the time it takes to bathe and skinbrush, and to cleanse and moisturize the face in the morning and the evening.

14-Day Personalized Care Chart

Major problems:

Moderate problems:

Minor problems:

If you have been using essential oils for many years, you will already appreciate how beneficial they can be to your health and well-being. If this is your first introduction to the wonderful world of aromatic oils, you have a pleasant surprise in store for you. During the next 14 days, you will be working hard to achieve your goals, but don't forget to enjoy the process. You are not just getting rid of problems, you are creating a foundation for future good health. And in the meantime, you are surrounding yourself with the uplifting and enriching fragrances of nature. Allow them to take you to a place of contentment so that your innate inner beauty can shine through.

To me, embarking on this 14-day aromabeauty plan can be likened to a DIY project for your home. While it requires energy, time and commitment, at the end of all the hard work and upheaval, you have improved the appearance and the comfort of your home, as well as its overall value. And you have something to be proud of, simply because you have done it yourself. Just as home improvements can correct the problems which, if neglected, would ultimately decrease the value of your home, by embarking on the 14-day aromabeauty plan, you will be able to correct those body problems which, if ignored, may ultimately exact a very high price in the form of ill health. When essential oils are used for aromabeauty, there is no such thing as 'just beauty care', as day by day you will be absorbing the healing and strengthening properties of the oils, which will not only transform your physical appearance, but improve the general state of your health. The 14-day aromabeauty plan is your personal DIY project, which can and will bring about a Dramatic Improvement in You.

Chapter 3

Creating a
home beauty spa

To create that dramatic improvement in you requires concentrated effort and willpower over a two-week period. This may sound like hard work but it should also be pleasurable in order to keep up your motivation and enthusiasm.

Pamper yourself by creating a beauty spa at home. Not only is it far more economical than enrolling at a health farm, it's infinitely more convenient. No need to cancel the milk, get a neighbour to feed the cats – not to mention the husband and the kids – or agonize over what to pack for two weeks. No one will be looking at you; no one will be judging. This is between you and your mirror. You and you alone are taking responsibility for correcting the problems that time and transgressions have accrued. There's no necessity to weigh yourself or wield the tape measure, or tick off a progress chart. Because you're in your own home, there's no restriction on food (but please make it healthy). It's your two weeks to work on yourself in private; once you see results then you can tell your friends.

I recommend setting aside a room, or a corner of a room, where you can store your oils and formulate your aroma-beauty preparations. Why not include a bowl of fresh flowers, a comfortable chair, a healing crystal or whatever makes you feel special. You need to lay out a selection of essential oils, good quality fatty oils and other items as listed below.

- nail brush
- large glass or china bowl for facial steaming

- kaolin/fuller's earth/green clay
- beeswax (from herb shops or hardware stores)
- honey (runny kind)
- friction strip – buy or make from old towel
- old sheet (cotton or wincyette) to protect furniture
- plastic sheeting (garden-shop type) or dustbin liners
- large and small towels
- old cotton sheet for body compress
- blanket for insulation
- cotton wool/cotton wool pads
- cling-film
- bottled water, such as Volvic or Evian
- empty ointment pots from a chemist

The essential oils needed will depend on which problem areas you choose to work on. There are a few oils, however, that are essential:

- juniper • lemongrass • orange • grapefruit • vetivert • lavender • myrtle

Your investment in these oils should last a long time. Essential oils are precious and only a few drops are needed at any time. Be sure to keep them tightly stoppered and away from sunlight as they are highly volatile. For this reason, only buy oils in dark bottles from a reputable supplier. While most suppliers are trustworthy, it is probably best to buy from a specialist source. It would be a shame to spend two weeks using inferior quality oils.

Almost as important as the quality of the essential oil is the quality of the fatty oil in which it is diluted. I recommend camellia, jojoba and sweet almond oil because, like essential oils, they penetrate the skin without leaving greasiness. You get what you pay for. Soyabean oil is very inexpensive, but it's really mainly produced for the 'fish and

chip' industry. Since many oils oxidize rapidly, it is important to use those fatty oils that are the most stable, such as
the ones I recommend. Sweet almond is available from
most chemists and jojoba from specialist suppliers. I am a
firm believer in the benefits of camellia since I first came
across it in Japan in 1989. It is not widely available at the
moment, and if you need a source of supply, please write to
me (see Addresses at the back of the book).

If you are on a budget or would prefer to build up your
stock of essential oils and other items more slowly, you
could consider sharing costs with a friend or two. For example, quarter of a bar of beeswax is all you'll need to make a
lip balm and a jar of daytime hand cream: the rest could be
shared with a friend or stored for later use and to make a
30ml bottle of **juniper blend** for the thighs requires only 5
drops juniperberry oil, 10 drops grapefruit oil, 3 drops
orange oil in 15ml of camellia and 15ml of jojoba.

Aromabeauty Products to Make in Advance

Before starting the 14-day aromabeauty plan it's a good idea
to make up a few of the recommended blends and products so that they are readily available, for example:

- Beeswax and jojoba hand cream
- Lip balm
- Vetivert in camellia
- Juniper blend
- Lemongrass blend
- Geranium blend
- Rose aromatic water
- Vetivert aromatic water
- Sandalwood aromatic water
- Lavender aromatic water
- Rose in camellia or jojoba

Ointment pots should be sterilized before use in the same way that jam jars are sterilized prior to making jam. Just wash them in soapy water, rinse well and stand upside down on a wire cake rack. Place the rack in a warm (not hot) oven at 120°C/250°F/gas mark ½, or the bottom oven of an Aga. Once dry, these pots are sterile but only if used straightaway. If left standing uncovered, bacteria from the air will find their way into your cream pots.

Vetivert in camellia

30ml camellia oil
1 drop vetivert oil
Mix in a tightly stoppered bottle. Tilt to mix.

This blend can be used for the thighs, face, elbows, hands , breasts, knees or buttocks.

Lemongrass blend

To a 30ml bottle add:
5 drops lemongrass
10 drops grapefruit
3 drops orange
15ml jojoba and 15ml camellia.

This blend can be used for the thighs, upper arms, elbows, ankles, knees, tummy and waist, chin or buttocks.

Juniper blend

To a 30ml bottle add:
5 drops juniper
10 drops grapefruit
3 drops orange

15ml jojoba and 15ml camellia

This blend can be used for the thighs, upper arms, tummy and waist, elbows, ankles, knees or buttocks.

Geranium blend

30ml camellia
4-5 drops geranium
6-7 drops ylang-ylang
Mix in a tightly stoppered bottle.

This blend can be used for the breasts, elbows or hands.

Rose in camellia

30ml camellia oil
5-10 drops rose oil (according to your preference)

This blend can be used for the breasts, shoulders, neck, solar plexus, face, or hands.

Rose in jojoba

30ml jojoba oil
5-10 drops rose
Mix in tightly stoppered bottle.

This blend can be used for the face, breasts, solar plexus, neck or hands.

Making your own aromatic waters

I do not use any alcohol for making aromatic waters because alcohol dissolves fats and robs the skin of the nutrients it needs to look healthy and young. Try putting some alcohol (gin or other spirit) on the back of your hand and see what effect it has.

Because cider vinegar helps viscous oils to dissolve, it becomes possible to make a wonderful variety of aromatic waters. Very thick oils such as sandalwood, vetivert and patchouli can now be incorporated into aromatic waters. Patchouli is best suited to teenage or greasy skins, sandalwood for dry skin and vetivert for mature skin. Mature means over 35 years old, as this seems to be the magic age when skin cell renewal noticeably slows down.

Rose aromatic water

4 drops rose absolute
1 small teaspoon cider vinegar
200ml spring water

Put 4 drops of rose into an empty glass bottle, add the cider vinegar and tilt bottle from side to side until the rose has mixed well in the vinegar, then top up with spring water leaving at least 1 inch (2.5 cm) free space between the top of liquid and bottle cap. Place lid on bottle and shake vigorously. You now have an astringent, antiseptic lotion which is inexpensive and extremely versatile. It needs to be shaken prior to use.

Rose aromatic water made with cider vinegar is gently astringent without being drying and is perfect for dehydrated skins where alcohol-based products should never be used.

This blend can be used for the face, hands, elbows or knees.

Vetivert aromatic water

4 drops vetivert
½ teaspoon cider vinegar
200ml spring water
Make up in same way as rose water.

This blend can be used for the face, elbows, neck, knees or hands.

Sandalwood aromatic water

4-6 drops sandalwood
½ teaspoon cider vinegar
200ml spring water
Make up in same way as **rose aromatic water**.

This blend can be used for the face, back, elbows, neck, knees or hands.

Patchouli aromatic water

3-4 drops patchouli
½ teaspoon cider vinegar
200ml spring water
Make up in same way as **rose aromatic water**.

This blend can be used for the face, hair, chest or shoulders.

Frankincense aromatic water

3-4 drops frankincense
½ teaspoon cider vinegar
200ml spring water
Make up in same way as **rose aromatic water**.

This blend can be used for the face, neck or hands.

Other essential oils which make beautifying aromatic waters and do not need the addition of cider vinegar – just a thorough shaking prior to use – include lavender, myrtle, lemon, clary sage, bergamot and orange.

Lavender aromatic water

2-4 drops lavender
200ml spring water
Shake well.

This blend can be used for the face, back, neck or hands.

Containers for aromatic waters

Many olive oil bottles are attractively shaped and corked, and when thoroughly washed with soapy water, make ideal containers for aromatic waters.

Spring water sold in half-litre bottles makes an alternative container for aromatic waters.

Making a lip balm

30g ointment pot (available from chemists)
¼ bar of beeswax, roughly chopped
3 tablespoons jojoba oil
Choice of essential oil (rose, geranium, sandalwood, lemon, orange, bergamot)

A sterile pot is important so prepare the pots before melting the ingredients (see page 21).

Place beeswax and jojoba in a bain marie (or a heatproof glass bowl that fits snugly over a small saucepan containing water). Place over a medium heat and allow to melt, stirring occasionally with a wooden skewer. Do not allow water to boil as steam or water could get into the mixture. When beeswax has completely melted into the jojoba, remove the bowl from the pan of water, wipe outside of bowl with tea towel and carefully pour the liquid into the prepared 30g pot. (Care must be taken to ensure that no water droplets go into the pot or the lip balm will be spoiled.) Add one or two drops of your chosen essential oil, stir mixture with wooden skewer and allow to cool naturally. When outside of pot is cool to the touch, screw on lid, and add a label. It is advisable to put the date on the label.

Making the daytime barrier cream

2 tablespoons jojoba/beeswax mixture (remains from
   making lip balm, see above)
3 tablespoons camellia oil
2 tablespoons hot water
4 drops of essential oil (choose from lavender, geranium,
   rose, sandalwood, patchouli, ylang-ylang, clary sage,
   myrtle, bergamot, frankincense, lemon, orange,
   vetivert, e.g. 2 drops patchouli + 2 drops geranium, or 2
   drops lavender + 2 drops clary sage)
2 x 60g ointment pots from chemist

Place jojoba/beeswax mixture in a heatproof bowl over a pan of hot water. When the mixture has melted, remove bowl from heat and allow to cool slightly (or transfer into another bowl). Add the hot water and whisk thoroughly (with hand or rotary whisk) until the ingredients have emulsified and the hand cream begins to resemble mayonnaise. Once you have an emulsion, add your choice of essential oils – for example, 2 drops geranium + 2 drops patchouli, or 3-4 drops myrtle oil – and whisk for a further 10 seconds. (It takes time to make an emulsion, so have patience.) Carefully

pour the mixture into sterile pots and allow to cool naturally. Do not be tempted to hurry the setting process by
standing the pots in a bowl of cold water as separation of oil
and water may occur with droplets of oil forming on the top
of the waxes. Separation of oils and water will also occur if
you have not beaten the mix until it has emulsified.

Setting the scene

Now you are ready to begin the 14-day aromabeauty plan.
Set the scene for your own private beauty spa. Make sure
the area you choose to work in is comfortably warm. You
want to get in touch with your body not your goosebumps!

Allow yourself the luxury of fluffy towels fresh from the
airing cupboard and put on your favourite background
music. Treat your sense of smell to the fragrance of essential
oils permeating the air.

For an uplifting mood, select oils such as clary sage, bergamot, geranium, grapefruit, frankincense, lemon, lemongrass, juniper, ravansara, rose, rosemary, orange,
sandalwood or ylang-ylang.

For a more relaxed atmosphere I suggest such oils as
geranium (neither completely sedative nor stimulant),
lavender, marjoram, myrtle, patchouli or vetivert.

Remember there's no place in this scene for stress and
hassle. Even if you are used to doing ten things simultane-
ously, now is your time to slow down and concentrate on *you*.

Chapter 4

Everyday beauty routine

By incorporting the use of essential oils into the daily routine of face care and hand care, our body is taking in small but regular amounts of essential oils which will help to keep us healthy and stress-free whilst strengthening the immune system – our friend, servant and security guard. Aromabeauty is not 'just' beauty care, even though our objective may be to improve the appearance of the face and hair. With nature's healing essential oils, the benefits go far beyond the surface layers of skin, interacting with us on a cellular level. When using essential oils for aromabeauty, we can truly experience the saying 'Beauty is more than skin deep'.

Although many of the regimes in this book will be more relevant to some people than others, and not everyone will want to work on a particular body area, there are a few tasks that we can all incorporate into our everyday life and allow the use of aromatic oils to become as routine as personal hygeine.

There is no recommended time for the everyday aromatic use. Just as with teeth cleaning, it takes as long as it takes. So when getting into the habit of cleansing and moisturizing the face with aromatic waters and oils, remember it takes whatever time is necessary, and whatever time you have available. Whether minutes or hours, your contact with aromatic oils will be enriching, health-promoting and beautifying.

Cleansing and moisturizing the face

The purpose of a moisturizer is twofold: to replenish the

skin with water, as water escapes from the skin's surface constantly throughout the day, and to protect the face from the worst effects of air-borne pollution and the harmful rays of the sun. If we merely applied water to the skin's surface it would quickly evaporate; for this reason we use an oil which locks the water into the skin.

Aromabeauty moisturizing uses pure and natural ingredients – oil and water – and creates very simple blends which need no emulsifiers or homogenisers. It is only when the water (in the form of an **aromatic water**) and the oil (in the form of an **oil blend**) are applied to the skin, that oil meets water.

Commercial moisturizing creams are little more than oil and water, held together in suspension by emulsifiers, homogenisers and kept germ-free and fresh by the addition of preservatives and anti-oxidents. Emulsifying agents are many and varied, and are derived from the animal, vegetable and mineral kingdoms. Isolated compounds such as polysorbates (and there are dozens of polysorbates) can be extracted from lauric acid (obtained from coconut oil), or be a condensate of sorbitol with the addition of stearic acid (found in butter, tallow and other animal fats in large quantities, and in small quantities in vegetable oils). To these ingredients add esters of p-hydroxybenzoic acid (a typical preservative) and we have a complex mixture of chemical isolates in a typical pot of commercial moisturizer, their only function being to prevent the oil and water from separating and to stop the mixture from becoming a breeding ground for micro organisms such as bacteria and fungi.

However, by mixing essential and fatty oils and waters on our skin, rather than in a pot, we can moisturize our complexions without any help from a scientific laboratory, and equally importantly, we can save a lot of money. All the **aromatic waters** and **oil blends** can be 'mixed and matched' throughout the book, and you will find that a bottle of **vetivert in camellia** can be used not only in combination

with an **aromatic water** to moisturize the face, but also for
breast care, hand care, and in the care of buttocks, knees
and elbows. A bottle of **aromatic water** such as **lavender
aromatic water** can be used with an **oil blend** to moisturize
the face, and can also be used to cleanse the skin by removing make-up, dirt and dead skin cells. A little **aromatic water**
on a cotton wool pad can also be used as an eye compress,
can tone and refresh the skin at any time of day, or can be
added to kaolin, fuller's earth or green clay to enhance the
healing and cleansing effect of a face mask. I cannot over-
emphasise the fact that **aromatic waters** are an integral part
of the aromabeauty plan for the face.

Instead of using a commercial moisturizing cream, try
the following.

In the morning

Any one of the numerous aromatic waters may be used for
morning face cleansing, with preference being given to
those waters best suited to your skin type. For example,
someone with dry skin may choose to cleanse her face with
vetivert aromatic water followed by moisturizing with a little
jojoba and **vetivert aromatic water**. Someone with greasy
skin may prefer a **patchouli aromatic water** or **lavender
aromatic water**. All skin types benefit from cleansing with
rose aromatic water. A morning face cleanse is important to
remove grease and dead skin cells which have accrued
overnight and to refresh the skin.

After cleansing , choose a combination of **aromatic water**
and an **oil blend** to moisturize the skin or, if you prefer,
simply apply a little jojoba. Making an aromatic moisturizer
is 'adult's play'. For example, using the **rose aromatic water**
and jojoba as a moisturizer, remove the lids from the **rose
aromatic water** and jojoba bottles, place the palm of your
hand on the jojoba bottle and invert it. To this little circle of
oil add a few drops of rosewater (just pour some from the

bottle onto your palm), place your other hand on top and mix together. Distribute evenly over your face, gently rub in and leave for a few minutes. Before applying make-up, tissue off any excess 'moisturizer', especially at the sides of nose. Jojoba oil, from the Arizona desert, is one of the world's finest natural emollients, and has a sun protection factor of 4. Combined with a few drops of homemade **rose aromatic water**, it provides an effective yet inexpensive, protective facial moisturizer. Jojoba and **rose aromatic water** are easily absorbed, leaving your skin smooth to the touch and delicately scented.

In the evening

Removal of make-up along with dirt accumulated throughout the day is the purpose of the evening face cleanse. It may be necessary to use a fatty oil to remove heavy make-up, followed by a refreshing cleanse with a cotton wool pad, impregnated with an aromatic water, such as **lavender aromatic water**.

As with the morning moisturizing, nourish the skin by applying some **aromatic water** and some massage oil, mixed together in the palm of the hand before being spread across the face and neck. Gently massage oil into the skin until it is all absorbed.

Bathing

As stated previously, there is no minimum recommended time for beauty treatments. The same applies to aromatic baths – if you only have fifteen minutes to spare before rushing off to catch a train for work, then you have fifteen minutes. If you have plenty of free time and can spend longer in an aromatic bath, so much the better. Even fifteen minutes in a bath of aromatic water is beneficial not only to the skin and physical body but also to stimulate and clarify the brain – perfect for those days when the mornings come too early.

Water temperature should be comfortably warm, i.e. a little more than blood temperature. A too hot bath is debilitating and you will feel tired and relaxed. The prospect of a cool bath, although rousing and ideal for waking us up, is not very tempting to most people. A long, lingering aromatic bath offers an opportune moment to condition the hair by saturating it with an aromatic hair treatment oil and wrapping it in a towel (see Chapter 6).

To start the day

Morning bath

A morning bath is ideally suited to using those essential oils which are renowned for their energizing and invigorating properties. After having slept for six, seven or eight hours, it can take several hours before the body is fully awake and alert, as can be witnessed by the numbers of commuters snoozing on trains every morning. An aromatic morning bath can make us alert and ready for the day ahead.

The morning bath is also the perfect time to carry out skin brushing. Skin brushing stimulates the lymphatic system into working efficiently, and can create a free-flowing movement of lymph which has become slow, at the same time giving a boost to your energy levels. It also encourages your body to let go of poisonous wastes through the skin, which has an invigorating effect on the body. Without contributing to the profits of the coffee industry we have the means to 'wake ourselves up' in the morning. To start the day on the right footing and banish the 'Monday Morning Blues', take a 15-30 minute aromatic bath using any of the following essential oils and skin brush whichever part of the body you will be working on later that day. If, for example, you have puffy ankles and knees, and have planned to massage them in the evening, spend a few minutes brushing these areas along with the relevant lymph nodes (see Chapter 12).

My long-time favourite morning bath combination is rosemary and geranium, but there are many invigorating essential oils from which to choose.

Choice of oils for the morning bath

- Rosemary and geranium
- Lemon and orange
- Clary sage and geranium
- Ravansara and orange

The amount of essential oil used depends on skin sensitivity and preferred strength of aroma. As a rule, 6-10 drops of essential oil are used in a full bath.

After bathing and whilst the skin is still warm, apply a light coating of oil to any areas of dry skin. A favourite of mine is the exquisite **rose in camellia**, which is quickly absorbed into the skin leaving a subtle and delightful fragrance.

To end the day

Evening bath

Depending upon the time of the evening bath, the choice of essential oils will vary. If the bath is taken prior to dinner or going out for the evening, then the choice of fragrance and temperature will be similar to the morning bath. If, however, the evening bath is taken towards the end of the day, and you have been under stress and feeling tense, then the choice of essences should be those which are renowned relaxants and encourage sleep. Geranium is neither relaxing nor stimulant but balancing and harmonizing and can therefore be used at any time of day. Clary sage can also be used both morning and evening, and is especially useful if you are feeling a little depressed. Its euphoric action will allow you to let go of worldly problems and leave them outside the bedroom door.

Water temperature for an evening bath can be considerably warmer than for a morning bath, enabling muscles to relax and tension to be released. Hot water will make you feel relaxed and ready for sleep because of the rush of blood to the head. Skin brushing is stimulating, so anyone wishing to wind down and drop off to sleep quickly should only skin brush in the morning.

Choice of oils for the evening bath

- Clary sage and myrtle
- Rose and ylang-ylang
- Lavender and marjoram
- Lavender and myrtle
- Myrtle and rose

Very viscous essential oils such as patchouli, sandalwood and vetivert do not lend themselves for use in the bath because the thickness of the oil prevents it from being able to disperse in the bathwater. To counter this problem, dissolve viscous oils in either a thin oil such as myrtle or lavender for example, or use a little cider vinegar. Cider vinegar does not emulsify the oils, but dissolves them. To an empty bottle add about 6 drops of the viscous oil. Add ½ teaspoon cider vinegar and top up with water. Shake vigorously before adding to bathwater.

Instant bathtime facial

Steam and oil are good companions and whilst taking your aromatic bath, the steamy air can open your pores and make dry skin even more receptive to nourishment and moisture. Before getting into a bath, thoroughly cleanse your face and apply a liberal coating of facial massage oil.

Slip into the fragrant water and soak up the luxurious atmosphere. After the bath simply tissue off the excess oil from your face and your skin will be moisturized and ready for the day or evening ahead – a wonderful time-saver when in a rush and there is not much time for skin care.

A glass of water taken before and after the bath will moisturize your skin from the inside.

Hand care

Hands and face are the two areas of our body most often exposed to the elements and, whilst we protect our facial skin with moisturizers and make-up, our hands are often neglected and become damaged. As there is only a thin layer of flesh over the bones of the hand, the skin on the backs of the hands can age more quickly than the skin of the face, and even if we are blessed with a youthful face, our hands can instantly reveal our true age. There are two ways to improve the condition of the hands:

1. A protective/barrier cream to be applied frequently during the day.
2. Nightly moisturizing with **oil blends** and **aromatic waters**.

Daytime barrier cream

A barrier cream has two functions. One is to provide an invisible film or barrier to our environment, the weather, central heating, water in all its usages – washing up, washing our hair, handling the laundry, etc. The second is to soften and moisturize dry skin and to feed it with nourishing fatty oils and essential oils.

Beeswax, jojoba oil, camellia oil, water and essential oils are all the ingredients necessary to make an emollient and protective hand cream which is also very cheap. Being simple to make, and not containing any preservatives, it is preferable to make up a batch every few weeks, rather than mix a large quantity at one time.

There is a huge range of essential oils which, although beneficial for the health of the skin, could be chosen merely for their fragrance, and which can be enhanced when two essential oils are carefully blended, for example lemon with orange, bergamot with orange, geranium with clary sage. Warm, earthy aromas make a pleasing bouquet when blended – vetivert with rose, patchouli with ylang-ylang, sandalwood with lavender. The final choice rests with you as the fragrance has to be agreeable to you if you are to apply it regularly throughout the day. See page 26 for instructions for making the daytime barrier cream.

Approximately two pots of hand cream can be obtained from the given quantities – and for very little expense. Keep one in the kitchen for use as a barrier cream before washing up, as well as for moisturizing hands afterwards. A second jar of hand cream could be kept in the bathroom to use every time you wash your hands.

Night time rejuvenating hand massage

Having experimented with various combinations of fatty oils and waxes, essential oil blends and **aromatic waters**, the combination which I find to be most effective is **vetivert in camellia oil** and **sandalwood aromatic water**.

Massage the hands before going to bed using **vetivert in camellia**. Hold your left hand with your right, and with right thumb massage the back of the hand, using small circular movements and working between the carpels (bones). Take one finger of your left hand between fingers and thumb of right hand and massage the entire length of finger. Rub your palms together and smooth the oil into the entire hand and wrist. Repeat on other hand. Next, take some **sandalwood aromatic water** and pour a little into the palm of one hand. Carefully rub into both hands, as if you were washing your hands. When dry, apply a little more **vetivert in camellia** and a little more **sandalwood aromatic water**. Keep applying a little more of these lotions until your hands cannot absorb any more. A pair of cotton gloves, if worn all night, will help with the penetrating action of the treatment which is guaranteed to soften and improve the condition of even the most 'taken for granted' hands.

The importance of patience

Tempting as it may be to try everything at once, I must advise a certain amount of caution and patience. Rome wasn't built in a day – and if it had been, it would probably have collapsed due to hurried, second rate workmanship.

There are several reasons why we should not attempt too much too soon.

Massage releases toxins from the tissues, especially the tissues of the arms, legs and buttocks – areas which have given shelter to unwanted body wastes and other poisons. As toxins are released, they must be eliminated from the body via the lymphatic system, blood stream, kidneys, bladder and digestive system. Sometimes, too, the process of elimination will cause spots and blemishes to appear on the surface of the skin where treatment is being given. Whichever route is used in the elimation process, it must be encouraged to flow at a steady pace. If too many toxins are released into the body's circulation at the same time, too great a strain can be put on the organs of elimation. This can result in toxins either being reabsorbed into the body again, or being unable to be eliminated quickly, circulating in the bloodstream and possibly resulting in nausea and headache, which can make you feel as though you are suffering from 'food poisoning'. You are actually suffering from a poisoning, but a poison which has been in the body for an unspecified length of time. It is not a serious problem, and anyone who has undertaken a fast will appreciate that the initial discomfort is short-lived as long as adequate water is consumed throughout the day. The lymph nodes can also become congested, just as the plughole in the kitchen sink will become blocked if we try to wash away too many tea leaves at one time. It then becomes necessary to use large quantities of water to disperse the blockage.

Perhaps you are a superwoman with unlimited amounts of energy, and the ability to tackle monumental tasks, but for mere mortals such as I, too much strain is rather offputting. Each task needs patience and time, in order for the massage oils to penetrate and for the massage to be effectively carried out. Good results come from hard work – and hard work is tiring but the good news is that hard work also burns up calories. If we attempt to do too much in one day we may become very tired – primarily the fingers and wrists which are doing most of the massage work, but also the biceps and triceps of the upper arms. If we overstrain ourselves and become exhausted we may not want to continue with a daily regime and therefore the possibility of reaching a pleasing and visible improvement at the end of the fourteen days could become a one-day aborted effort. Or we may decide that we are going to tackle all of our problem areas in a day, because perhaps we have a whole day free to ourselves, but then find that tasks are skimped in the rush to tackle the next one.

For all of these reasons, it is advisable to be realistic about what can be accomplished each day. Massage of the thighs, buttocks, or whichever area, is tiring at first and for a few days your fingers may ache a little. However, just as a concert pianist or typist is able to use their fingers for long periods of time, you will find that with regular use you will be able to massage your problem areas for longer and longer periods without experiencing any discomfort.

Chapter 5

The Face

The problems: Dry and dehydrated skin; greasy skin; maturing skin; lifeless skin; teenage skin; double chin; after-effects of spots on chin; tired and irritated eyes; crow's feet; thin eyelashes; dry and chapped lips.

The causes: Lack of natural oils or excess secretion of sebum; insufficient water; smoking; lack of nourishment (inside and out); polluted environment; sun.

The solutions: Massage oils to feed and nourish the skin; rehydration of the skin with aromatic waters and rebalancing oils; cleansing; rejuvenating (face lift) massage; friction massage; facial masks and facial steaming; cleansing regime for teenage skin; decongesting oils; soothing aromatic compresses; toning the eye area; nourishing oils for lashes and brows; softening and protecting lip balms.

Care of the face

Your face may not launch a thousand ships, nor be your fortune, but it is the part of you that is presented to the world. Although there is a saying 'don't judge a book by its cover', in reality we are often judged by the look of our face. Whether in our opinion we are beautiful, attractive or plain, if we are feeling unhappy or under emotional stress, it can be seen in our faces. The mind is mirrored in the face and when mentally stressed, our skin can lose its attractiveness. When we feel happy and contented, a certain 'glow' comes from within, which not only makes us feel good but is visible to others.

The skin is a living organ and the largest of the body's organs. It is composed of three main layers, although the only part we see is the dead layer. When we apply massage oils to the top layer, the epidermis, the tiny molecules of essential oil penetrate to the dermis (or corium) where the elasticity of the skin is governed. It is in this layer that fibres of collagen, elastic fibres and fibres of connective tissue are intermingled, and it is the alignment of these fibres that gives skin its elasticity. Also in this layer are the hair roots, glands, blood vessels and lymph vessels. A complex structure indeed, which gives us the word 'complexion'.

The epidermis itself is divided into three main layers – the top, visible layer which is keratinized, a lower layer where plump cells become flatter and harder, and the basement layer (or basal layer) where skin cells are generated (see Figure 1). Our skin is constantly renewing itself and it takes about 30 days for a newly formed skin cell to move step-by-step through the layers of the epidermis until it becomes cornified and stratified (hard and flat) and eventually is rubbed off the surface. Vitamin A controls the rate of cornification and anyone suffering from a Vitamin A deficiency will have hard, horny skin.

Figure 1. The skin

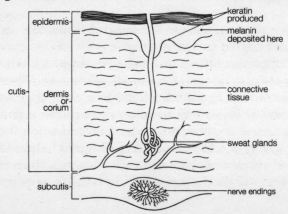

Healthy cells can prevent harmful substances from entering them, and as well as receiving nutrients from an adequate diet, cells can be strengthened from the outside, by the application of essential oils to the skin.

Essential oils, because of their concentrated strength, must *always* be diluted in water or oil before using on the face. There is a large choice of fatty oils available for a facial massage oil – avocado, sweet almond, grapeseed, corn oil, soya bean, peanut, sesame, olive, safflower, sunflower, walnut, camellia – and in theory, any oil would suffice to dilute the essential oils. However, the skin is being fed from the outside and these fatty oils vary enormously in their benefits to the skin. For example, if we compare camellia oil and soya bean oil, it is like the difference between a healthy nutritious meal and a junk food snack. See Compendium: Part B for a chart listing their different properties.

One of the most important factors for me is the stability of the fatty oil I am using. When a fatty oil begins to oxidize, free radicals are formed which, when applied to the body, can damage the skin cells and do nothing to increase the cell's strength. Camellia oil does not oxidize, and I have absolute confidence in using it for the care of my face. It penetrates very quickly, without leaving any greasiness and imparts a satin-soft sheen. It is the perfect accompaniment to pure essential oils. Why put expensive, beautiful essences into a base oil such as soya bean or safflower oil which is only fit to be used in the chip shop? Jojoba is an oil (or rather a liquid wax) that I also use extensively for skin care. Like camellia, it does not oxidize, but leaves a beautiful texture to the skin and gives a light, luminous appearance.

Everyday the skin sheds its outer cells and new skin cells are given life, so we need to cleanse and massage the face everyday, giving Mother Nature a really good helping hand. Chapter 4 provides a daily skincare routine, whilst in this chapter you will find more specific tasks to improve the

appearance of your skin, the look of your face and ultimately your overall well-being.

Dry and dehydrated skin

There are many essential oils which, when blended together
and incorporated into a fatty base oil, make wonderful
massage oils. We can create blends to feed, regularize, moisturize, rejuvenate ageing skin, or bring antiseptic healing
powers to troubled skin.

It is not strictly necessary to make a complex blend of
essential oil and fatty oils , and a highly effective massage oil
for dry and dehydrated skin could simply be **vetivert in
camellia**. For some skin problems, the massage is as important as the blend of oils used.

Facial masks and facial steaming are necessary for some
skin types and specific conditions, but are of secondary
importance to the basic feeding and moisturizing of the
skin with aromatic oils and waters.

Vetivert in camellia

Vetivert oil is very important in skincare as it encourages
the tissues to retain water. Loss of moisture is one of the
main factors in ageing skin and occurs as we get older
because body tissues do not replenish themselves as they
did in our youth. Vetivert has a very powerful (some would
say overpowering) aroma, and should be used in very dilute
form. Only one drop is needed in 30ml of camellia oil, or
three drops to a 100ml bottle. There are several ways in
which I use **vetivert in camellia**.

1. As a face massage oil at the end of the day.
2. Combined with **rosewater** as an effective morning
   moisturizer.
3. For breast care, with or without the additon of

geranium and ylang- ylang essential oils.
4. As a massage oil for thighs, knees and buttocks after using the **lemongrass blend** or **juniper blend**.
5. In combination with **rosewater** or **sandalwood aromatic water** for nightly hand massage.

Greasy skin

Greasy skin is only a problem after the onset of puberty, and before this turning point in our lives, the majority of us have smooth childhood skin. At birth we have approximately 100 sebaceous (oil-producing) glands on every square centimetre of our skin with the exception of the soles of the feet, palms of the hands and the eardrum, but immediately after birth these glands become dormant and only become active again at the onset of puberty. On some areas of the body the concentration of sebaceous glands is much more intense – up to 900 per square centimetre on the face, scalp, forehead and genital region.

Our sebaceous glands produce a thick, oily, colourless secretion produced in cells or lobes, which break down and empty their contents in ducts which in turn empty into hair follicles. The lifespan of each one of these lobes is only about a week, but is an ongoing process which lubricates our skin continually.

The content of sebum is a very complex mix of hundreds of fatty acids; a significant proportion of them being the well-known fatty acids palmitic, myristic, stearic, oleic and linoleic. It is the secretion of sebum onto the skin of the face and scalp that can become a problem for teenagers and older women alike as the face looks shiny, make-up runs, the presence of surface oil can cause blocked pores which attract dirt (blackheads), and infection of the ducts by micro-organisms can produce pimples or acne.

Thorough cleansing of the skin is of vital importance, and

when carried out several times a day using **aromatic waters**, will prevent a build-up of sebum on the skin's surface. Facial steaming and the use of clay masks can be very helpful in keeping the complexion clear and blemish-free, and should include one of the following essential oils: bergamot, lemon, myrtle, lavender, geranium, patchouli, ylang-ylang.

Both cleansing with **aromatic waters** and using an aromatic facial steam bring the skin into contact with a very small amount of essential oil, which has beneficial results, but to treat a blemished complexion, it is necessary to apply a stronger concentration of essential oils in a fatty oil base. You may wonder why a fatty oil is being used on skin which is already greasy, and the answer is two-fold. Firstly, essential oils are far too concentrated to be used neat, and must always be diluted before applying to the skin and, as essential oils dissolve in fatty lipids, the preferred medium for dilution is a fatty oil. The second reason is that, as fatty oils contain lipids in much the same way as the skin and we know that essential oils dissolve easily in fatty oils, we know also that essential oils will dissolve into the oil secreted by the sebaceous glands. When an essential oil, such as bergamot, is massaged into the face, its antiseptic properties seep down into the deeper layers of the skin to kill bacteria, thus protecting and healing the skin and preventing infection.

A simple recipe for a nightly massage is 2 drops of any one of the above essential oils plus 1 teaspoon of good quality fatty oil or jojoba.

Of great value to the skin, due to their super-absorbency, are the fatty oils of jojoba and camellia. Camellia oil is very high in oleic acid (92%) which makes it very stable – that is, it does not oxidize. If a cheap oil such as safflower is used as a base for essential oils, the beneficial effects of the essences may be hindered by the presence of free radicals, formed by the oxidation of the fatty oil. Other recommended fatty oils with high levels of oleic acid include the strong-smelling virgin olive oil, containing 72% oleic acid, and the almost odourless sweet almond oil, containing 70% oleic acid. Jojoba oil is a liquid wax which does not oxidize, and which has super-emollient properties.

Whichever oils you choose for the care of your skin, the blend should be massaged into the face, forehead (right up to the hairline) and chin immediately after the night time face cleansing routine with an **aromatic water**, such as **patchouli aromatic water**.

Facial steaming

Spotty and greasy skins will benefit most from a facial steam once or twice a week incorporating a healing, antiseptic essential oil such as myrtle. Young 'problem' skins also benefit from a facial steam once or twice a week, alternating with a facial mask on other nights.

Dry or dehydrated skins can be moisturized by the use of a fortnightly facial steam. However, anyone with delicate skin which is prone to broken veins should avoid facial steaming, as the hot moisture causes blood to rush to the skin's surface, further weakening the capillary walls.

Preparing a facial steam

To a large glass bowl, salad bowl (not wooden) or mixing bowl, add 1 pint boiled water and a cup of cold water. The water must not be boiling when the essential oil is added or the essence will evaporate too readily. If the steam is still too intense for your comfort, add a little more cold water. Add three drops of myrtle or lavender to the water's surface, drape a towel over your head and position your face over the steaming bowl. Be careful not to put your nose too close to the hot water. Hot water can be dangerous, so please make sure that pets and small children are not around.

Mature skin

Rejuvenating the face

Almost all aromatherapists insist that facial massage should be of the lightest possible strokes for fear of stretching the delicate tissues of the skin. It is true that an acneic skin should be handled with care so that neither the spread of infection nor bruising to an already damaged skin occurs, and women with delicate skin or broken veins should treat their skin gently. But I have to disagree with the general assumption that our faces need to be treated like Dresden china.

My research has shown me that anyone with normal, dry or ageing skin can benefit greatly from a friction massage. During one of my forays through the British Library I came across a book *Old Age* written in 1912 by a gentleman called Sanford Bennett. He was a firm believer in the restorative and rejuvenating powers of friction massage and photographs of him bear testimony to his beliefs. These photographs show how his regime so rejuvenated his skin that when he was in his seventies he looked far younger than when in his fifties. Sanford Bennett did not believe in the use of any beauty products for the skin, and relied upon facial exercises and massage of the skin. I was so amazed I duly set about proving his theories on myself.

As a firm believer in the benefits of aromatherapy oils for beauty care, I have expanded upon Sanford Bennett's friction massage and incorporate the use of essential oil blends and aromatic waters into my rejuvenating friction massage. Giving your face a friction massage has many benefits: it tones the underlying muscles, keeping them in good shape; it nourishes the skin by bringing blood to the surface, thereby allowing dietary nutrients to be made available for cell renewal; it rubs away dead skin cells, which helps to make the complexion look lighter and more youthful; and it prepares the skin to receive the **aromatic waters**. By doing the friction massage two or three times a week, it is possible to improve the youthfulness of the face dramatically in a relatively short period of time. In fact, this potent combination is probably as good as a face lift.

Rejuvenating friction massage

Secure hair back from forehead and liberally spread jojoba or camellia oil over the face, from the hairline down to the chin. Work on one section of the face at a time. Tense the muscles (as a man does when shaving) so that the skin is not pulled and stretched. Starting with one section (say the left cheek) press and rotate the skin and underlying muscles, using the first three fingers of the left hand. Feel for any sore areas, and gently but firmly massage these areas until the skin begins to feel hot. Next, put your right thumb inside your mouth so that the pad of the thumb is pressing against the inside of the cheek. Squeeze flesh between thumb and fingers and move the thumb in tiny circular movements so that all of the fleshy inside cheek has been massaged. Repeat these movements on the right side of the face. Next, place your palms of hands onto your cheeks (see figure 2) and with facial muscles tensed, buff the cheeks with circular movements. Massage of the forehead follows, and in order to tense the muscles it is simplest to close the eyes tightly, and then to buff the skin with the palm of one hand. Begin in the centre of the forehead, and with a circular motion, work outwards towards the temples. Before massaging the chin, place the lips together so that lips are not visible (as we do to spread lipstick evenly after application), and with the palms of hands, buff the skin. Move your mouth (again, as a man does when shaving) so that there is always enough muscle tension, and massage in this way around the mouth, so that tiny lines are encouraged to disappear.

After the massage apply a little aromatic water (such as **rose aromatic water**), followed by a coating of **vetivert in camellia**, and finally another generous application of **rose aromatic water**. The rejuvenating friction massage is very stimulating to the skin, and perfectly prepares it to absorb aromatic waters and massage blends. You could of course make your own massage blend with a choice of essential oils, but because of the intensity of the massage, I prefer to follow the massage with simple but effective blends.

With the rejuvenating friction massage there are two important rules to remember. One is that the skin must first be well lubricated with a good fatty oil, and the second is that the facial muscles must be tensed before massaging. This is very important to observe as the facial skin should not be stretched or pulled whilst it is in a relaxed state.

I recommend that this rigorous face massage be used between one and three times a week, but you should be sensitive to your own skin's needs. Thread veins on the cheeks may become slightly worse at first, but after a few days the walls of the capillaries will begin to get stronger by the astringent action of the rose and the fresh supplies of blood being brought to the surface of the skin. (Consumption of alcohol increases the problem of thread veins, as alcohol causes the capillaries to soften and expand.)

Sallow lifeless skin

Hyperaemic oils

An alternative to the very popular (but often hazardous) skin-peeling – whether fruit acid or chemical in action – is to massage the face with a hyperaemic blend of essential oils. Hyperaemia means to bring a rush of blood deliberately to the skin's surface, causing localized heat. Myrtle is my first choice of hyperaemic oils for use in facial care.

Myrtle can be applied to the face in several ways – in a face mask, a massage oil, or a facial steam. To really 'buck up' skin which has been neglected for a long time or damaged by cigarette smoking, I recommend that the face is treated daily to either a five minute facial steam, a fifteen minute face mask or a ten minute massage using 3 drops of myrtle to every teaspoon camellia oil.

Fruit acid peeling works by removing the top layer of skin so that the face looks younger, but unless skilfully executed, the procedure can remove more than just the top layer of skin and there is a danger that skin can become damaged – tantamount to a burn. The quest for beauty does not have to involve such risks.

Simple friction massage

An alternative to using a hyperaemic massage oil to replace

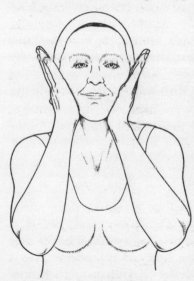

a sallow complexion with a glowing healthy skin is to buff the face with the palms of the hands, so that the friction brings a rush of blood to the skin's surface. Firstly apply a coating of jojoba or camellia oil to the face, and position hands on cheeks (see figure 2). Using the flat of the fingers and the palms of the hands, lightly rub the surface of your skin using circular movements, rather like the way a child washes his face. Buff the skin until it feels quite warm to the touch and then apply any of the aromatic waters, patting the fragrant

Figure 2. Friction Massage

water into the skin until it will absorb no more.

Regime for a teenage skin

Pimples can be treated kindly by cleansing at least twice a day with an **aromatic water**. Essential oils not only clean the skin but are antiseptic, thereby killing surface bacteria. They also leave behind a fine layer of healing essence to give further protection.

Aromatic water for teenage skins

Sometimes teenagers with spotty skins use alcohol-based facial lotions believing that the alcohol will dry up the excess grease and shrivel up the spots. The effect is a temporary tightening of the skin's surface and therefore a clamping down of the oil ducts, but soon the body will again secrete oil – possibly more than previously! Essential oils such as patchouli, myrtle, lavender and bergamot are cleansing and antiseptic. Cider vinegar is gently astringent and contains many vitamins and minerals. Combined in an aromatic face-wash, this simple and inexpensive lotion cleanses the skin, killing bacteria and leaving a thin protective film on the surface. Cider vinegar serves two purposes. Firstly, it dissolves the essential oil and helps its dispersal in the water, and secondly it can restore skins that have been damaged by washing with alkali soaps, to a healthy pH balance.

Face mask for a teenage skin

Pimples respond particularly well to a regular face mask. The easiest and cheapest bases to obtain are kaolin, which is a fine white clay, or fuller's earth powder. Whichever one you choose, place two or three heaped teaspoons into a small bowl, add 3 drops of myrtle oil and enough home-made **rose aromatic water** to mix it to a spreadable consistency. Spread all over the skin of the face, avoiding the eye area, nostrils and mouth, and allow to dry. The mask may be left on a spotty or greasy skin longer than on a dry or normal skin, but the length of time should be determined by you. If the mask is left on the skin until it dries out, it draws more impurities from the skin which is beneficial for greasy, blemished skin, but even if only left on the face for 5-10 minutes, its astringent and 'drawing' action will stimulate the circulation whilst removing sebum, dirt and poisons from the skin. Used regularly, the myrtle mask will quickly bring about a noticeable improvement in the complexion. The mask is rinsed off with cotton wool and cold running water. Pat face dry with a clean towel or face flannel and whilst skin is damp, apply a little jojoba oil with a drop of lavender, bergamot or geranium, or alternatively use a little Vitamin E oil. Massage gently into the skin, leave for a few minutes and blot off any excess oil with a tissue.

Emergency pimple treatment

Pimples should never be squeezed when they are small red bumps because at this stage there is nothing to remove and you will only cause bruising of the tissues. However, when a pimple has come to a head you have a choice of whether to dab it with neat lavender or tea tree, or to squeeze the spot. Most beauty books advise against squeezing spots but if carried out very carefully you can quickly and efficiently rid your body of waste matter. If you choose the latter (because you are going somewhere special and you feel self-conscious about the 'mountain' on your chin), then very carefully set about removing it. A sharp needle should be sterilized by first wiping with a piece of cotton wool moistened with one drop of lavender. Gently prick the spot with the needle – not downwards into the spot, but sideways so that the tip of the needle is parallel with the face. With clean cotton wool, apply sufficient pressure to discharge the accumulated debris (a mixture of bacteria and dead lymph cells) and finally, dab the area with one of the antiseptic oils – lavender, tea tree, niaouli, ravansara, juniper, lemon, myrtle or berg-amot. It may sting for a few seconds but it will prevent a spread of infection. If at all possible, do not apply make-up for the next 24 hours. An alternative to squeezing is to facial steam the complexion at the first signs of a spot. The hot, moist vapours combined with antiseptic and healing aromas, promote elimination through the skin and help to unblock clogged pores – often the cause of blackheads and spots.

Face masks

A face mask is one of the fastest and simplest means of revi-talizing the facial skin. A clay mask is deep-cleansing, draw-ing impurities from the skin, and is of considerable benefit to anyone prone to spots, blackheads or blocked pores. Clay masks, when drying out, remove dead skin cells from the face, leaving a glowing, vital complexion.

Clay mixes very well with **aromatic waters** and essential oils and the permutations are endless, making it fun to create your own combination. Whatever your skin type, a clay mask should not be used too frequently. Greasy skins could use a face mask three times a week. Blemished skins can be treated to a mask every other day. A sallow, lifeless complexion will benefit from a twice-weekly clay mask. All other skin types should not use a clay mask more than once a week.

Three different clays for masks

Kaolin
The use of kaolin clay will give you a white face mask. This clay is very fine and because of its absorbency, has long been used in combination with morphine as primary care for diarrhoea. Classified by the British Pharmacopeia as being pure enough to use as a medicine, kaolin is a safe and soothing base for a facial mask. Can be used on any skin

type and is especially suited to dry or mature skins. One tablespoon of kaolin will thicken with 7.5ml water.

Green clay
Readily available in France, it is difficult to obtain in the UK, although a few mail order companies offer green clay. Not as fine as kaolin yet lighter than fuller's earth, green clay is suitable for all skin types. One tablespoon green clay will thicken with 10ml water.

Fuller's earth
Widely available, this clay is brownish-green in colour and dries to a dark green finish. Originally used by the textile industry for cleaning and fulling woollen cloth – hence the name 'fuller's earth'. It mixes very easily with water and essential oils, and is ideal for frequent use by teenagers or anyone plagued by spots or greasy skin. One tablespoon fuller's earth will thicken with 12.5-15ml water.

Making a fuller's earth mask

2 level tablespoons fuller's earth powder
½ teaspoon runny honey
2 drops essential oil
sufficient water to mix a smooth yet thick consistency

Choose an essential oil according to your skin type. Myrtle is ideal for spotty skins as well as for grey, lifeless skin; lemon for greasy skin; lavender or rose for mature skin. However any of the following oils may also be used in face packs: niaouli, bergamot, clary sage, frankincense, geranium, patchouli, sandalwood, tea tree, ylang-ylang.

Place powder in a small bowl, add honey and essential oil to bowl and enough water to achieve a smooth but thick consistency. If the mask seems too thick, just add a little more water – literally a few drops at a time until you have the desired consistency. If the mask seems too thin, add a little more powdered clay. Mix to a smooth paste and spread the mask over the face, forehead and chin, avoiding the eyes and lips. Leave on for at least 5 minutes.

With a large swab of cotton wool and lots of running water, remove all traces of mask. Pat dry and apply a little jojoba oil (for normal, greasy or spotty skin) or rosehip seed oil or Vitamin E oil (for dry or wrinkled skin). Thirty minutes later, apply a liberal coating of jojoba and then pat on some **rose aromatic water**. The skin will look and feel fresh, younger and clearer, with a more refined texture. This is a simple yet effective recipe, guaranteed to revitalize and moisturize the complexion.

Instant face mask

2 teaspoons kaolin, fuller's earth or green clay
Sufficient liquid – **sandalwood aromatic water** or **patchouli aromatic water** – to mix to the required consistency.

If the mixture has a consistency of cream, you may apply one coat, allow to dry out slightly and then apply a second coat to problem areas such as the chin and sides of the nose. Kaolin is a very fine powder and makes a thinnish mask. Fuller's earth is very absorbent and it is possible to apply a thick coating of mask to the skin. Green clay can be applied moderately thickly.

Remove mask with large pieces of cotton wool and lots of cold water. When all traces of mask have been removed and the skin is still damp, massage in some jojoba oil or a little of the **vetivert blend**.

Tightening facial mask

1 egg white, size 3
1 drop rose oil

Place egg white in a bowl and whisk with rotary or hand whisk until frothy. Add 1 drop rose oil and whisk for a further 10 seconds. Apply mask all over face and neck (with a pastry brush, cotton wool pad or fingertips), paying particular attention to areas of the face prone to wrinkles, such as the forehead and around the eye sockets. Leave on the face for 5-10 minutes, until skin feels taut. Remove with cotton wool pads moistened with water. The skin should feel smooth and silky. Whilst skin is still damp take a small amount of rosehip seed oil or Vitamin E oil and work into the face, neck and forehead with fingertips, going right up to the hairline. Do not apply to the skin directly under the eye, but dot it onto the laughter lines (crow's feet) at the outer edges of the eye.

The chin

Double chin

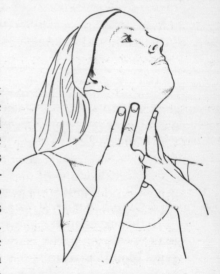

Lemongrass would not normally be used on the face as it is very powerful and could irritate the delicate skin of the face. However, because of its remarkable ability to decongest the tissues by burning up toxins in the connective tissues I like to use it under the chin. This helps reduce a double chin, an area where fat can accumulate easily and where toxins can lodge.

Figure 3. Double chin massage

Apply **lemongrass blend** (or jojoba if preferred) to the underside of the chin and tilt head back so that the skin of the neck is taut. Using only the tips of the first two fingers of each hand, slide fingertips along jaw line until they reach the angle of the jaw. Repeat several times. Position the same fingers just under jawbone in centre of chin and gently stroke the 'double chin', drawing the fingers down the neck towards the cervical lymph nodes. (See Figure 3). Continue this gentle stroking of the under-chin area and be sensitive to any lumps and bumps that may be under the skin's surface. Gently massage these toxic and stagnant spots to encourage them to disperse and immediately after working on this area, spend a few moments massaging the lymph nodes involved with the drainage of fats and toxins from the head and neck (see Figure 4).

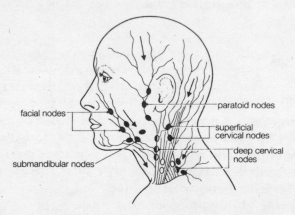

Figure 4. Lymph nodes of the face and neck

If the skin under the chin is very loose and flabby, massage the area with **vetivert in camellia** instead of **lemongrass blend**, as vetivert has the ability to attract and retain moisture in the underlying tissues of the skin, making the flesh look plumper.

After-effects of spots

Even in our thirties or forties, our chin may still bear the after-effects of teenage spots that have been squeezed and, as the chin has only a thin covering of muscle and fat, it is more difficult to heal itself than more fatty areas such as the cheeks. **Lemongrass blend** can be used on this localized area, as its ability to clear toxins from the connective tissue will help to restore a smooth appearance to the chin.

Apply **lemongrass blend** to the chin, from under bottom lip (avoiding the lip) to the tip of the chin. With second finger of right hand, massage in small circular movements whilst immobilizing the skin with two fingers of the left hand. Firmly, but without being rough, work this area for 5-10 minutes.

The eyes

As the whole body becomes less toxic and the metabolism is improved, eyes will automatically become clearer. Working on the lymphatic nodes, both with skin brushing and massage, toxins which may have rested in the body for years are encouraged to go. As the liver is better able to cleanse the blood, the kidneys to eliminate poisons, and the skin works optimally to eliminate waste matter through its surface, there will be a significant improvement in the colouring of the skin under the eyes.

Tired, irritated eyes

Tired eyes that feel sore and eyes irritated by cigarette smoke, wind, central heating, etc, can be quickly soothed with an aromatic eye compress. A piece of cotton wool or a cotton wool pad is saturated with **lavender aromatic water** or other soothing **aromatic water**, such as **rose aromatic water**, the excess being squeezed out before the pad is applied to the eyes. Lie down for at least ten minutes whilst the compress is in place.

Crow's feet

To treat wrinkles of the delicate skin around the eye and tighten the skin, apply an egg white and rose oil mask. Whisk the egg white in a small bowl and when frothy add a drop of rose oil. Mix for a few seconds more and apply to the skin immediately around the eye socket. Upper eyelids and eyebrows may be included in this tightening mask. Allow to dry and rinse off with wet cotton wool pads. Whilst skin is still damp, apply a little rosehip seed oil or Vitamin E oil and gently pat into the skin at outer edges of eyes.

Thin eyelashes and eyebrows

When eyelashes have become thinned by constant wearing of mascara, give them a holiday from mascara and treat them instead to a coating of jojoba oil. Eyelashes, like the hairs on our head, are dead and therefore to apply jojoba on the tips only would do little good. Apply the jojoba as you would mascara, and also massage a little into the eyelid where the lashes spring forth. The skin surrounding the eye is very sensitive and feeding of the eyelashes should not be repeated too frequently. Once a week is ample.

If you have thin, straggly eyebrows and would like to try to improve their condition, rub a little jojoba oil along their length, as part of everyday aromabeauty.

The lips

Dry and chapped lips

Dry lips may occur when we are unavoidably outside on a windy day or when we have too much sun on our face. However, dry lips usually denote that we are not drinking enough water and are in fact a little dehydrated. Acknowledge this sign as our body's request for more water

Rejuvenating Face Plan

Day	1	2	3	4	5	6	7	8	9	10	11	12	13	14
Rejuvenating friction massage	✓			✓			✓			✓			✓	
Clay mask (followed by jojoba or Vitamin E oil)		✓												
Rose and egg white mask									✓					
Double chin massage	✓				✓				✓					✓
Chin massage (to remove scarring)				✓				✓				✓		
Eyelash treatment						✓							✓	

Sallow Skin Plan

Day	1	2	3	4	5	6	7	8	9	10	11	12	13	14
Facial steaming	✓			✓			✓			✓			✓	
Facial mask			✓			✓					✓			
Simple friction massage			✓		✓			✓			✓			✓

Teenage Skin Plan

Day	1	2	3	4	5	6	7	8	9	10	11	12	13	14
Cleanse 2-3 times a day	✓	✓	✓	✓	✓	✓	✓	✓	✓	✓	✓	✓	✓	✓
Face mask		✓		✓		✓			✓			✓		✓
Facial steam			✓					✓			✓			✓
Night massage oil (see page 44)	✓	✓	✓	✓	✓	✓	✓	✓	✓	✓	✓	✓	✓	✓

and drink an extra glass or two. To protect the lips from wind, sun and air pollution, throughout the day apply a little home-made beeswax and jojoba lip balm. Fragrance your lip balm sparingly with any one of the following essences: **rose, sandalwood, orange, lemon, bergamot, geranium**.

And finally...

Don't forget the value of 'beauty sleep' – it is not an old wives' tale that we need our sleep if we wish to be beautiful. The body repairs broken-down tissues and renews cells whilst we are asleep, which for most people is one third of every day. If we occasionally have to function on four, five or six hours a night, no irreparable damage will be done, but if we consistently work eighteen-hour days, or dance the night away, then we are denying our complexion, as well as our general health, the full benefit of the body's repair service. Sleep *is* important.

Chapter 6

Hair care
and head massage

The problems: Dry, lacklustre hair; dandruff; excess grease; hair loss; tension in head; stressed out feeling.

The causes: Lack of nourishment; external chemicals (hair dyes, perms); environment; sun; stress; bottling up emotions.

The solutions: Aromatic oils for hair treatments; hair shampoos and rinses; head and neck massage.

Healthy hair

The acquisition of beautiful, healthy hair is something almost all women aspire to. Whether school students or grannies, every woman recognizes that her hair is indeed 'her crowning glory'. But often, in the pursuit of a beautiful head of hair, we actually cause damage by seeking out the help of chemical products – to lighten, colour, curl, straighten – to change our hair into our perceived image of loveliness.

Our hair is only a collection of individual hairs – approximately 250,000 – each one rooted deep in the scalp, and just as dependent on good nutrition as the skin on any other part of our body. If we are not receiving the nutrients our body needs for proper maintenance, then we will not have a healthy skin from which the hair can grow. Each person's body is programmed to take and use daily dietary nutrients for the most vital functions of the body – to repair the heart tissue, liver cells, etc – and whatever is left over is available for use by the skin and hair. So if we are not eating healthy, cell-building foods we are likely to have skin and hair that is weak, lack-lustre and easily damaged. Our body is keeping us alive, first and foremost, and cannot spare the necessary nutrients to produce beautiful hair. Common sense in what we eat is the first step towards healthy, shining hair.

Even if our diet is sensible and nutritious, we may not benefit from the nutrients if our body is not absorbing vitamins and minerals from what we have eaten. Stress is one common reason why we sometimes fail to absorb sufficient goodness from our food. This is why, when someone is suffering badly from stress, their hair can start to thin and their skin may look as though they have suddenly 'aged'. Normal daily hair loss is between 50-100 hairs.

An individual hair grows at the rate of about 1cm per month, although some people's hair grows faster or slower than the average. My hair grows at the rate of 1.5cm a month, which I attribute to a healthy, mostly vegetarian diet and liberal use of essential oils – not only to feed and protect my skin, but to take away stress and tension from my body, allowing it to function normally.

When under stress our muscles tense up causing, amongst other problems, headaches and nausea. But beyond the noticeable physical symptoms, tension is also responsible for preventing the normal flow of blood, lymph, sebum and other nutrients. In effect, if we are really 'stressed out', we can literally be starving our hair to death. Massaging the head with essential oils in jojoba prevents premature hair loss in two ways. Firstly, the physical act of massaging the head will dispel tension caused by stress, whether emotional, mental or environmental, by relaxing the scalp and allowing the circulation of blood (which carries vitamins, minerals and proteins), lymph (which carries lymphocytes to the scalp, and carries away body wastes and toxins) and sebum (the body's own secretion of oil to lubricate the hair). Secondly, essential oils, when massaged into the scalp, will penetrate through the epidermis to the dermis and connective tissue. It is in the connective tissue that the hair 'bulb' is rooted (see Figure 5).

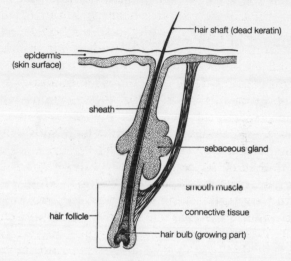

hair shaft (dead keratin)

epidermis
(skin surface)

sheath

sebaceous gland

smooth muscle

connective tissue

hair follicle

hair bulb (growing part)

Figure 5. The hair

Topically, there is much that we can do to improve the condition of the scalp – the flower bed or soil from which the hair blossoms. And just as we must feed the soil if we wish to produce beautiful roses, so it is with our scalp. One of the best 'foods' for hair and scalp is jojoba oil. A liquid wax from the deserts of Arizona, this plant has long and powerful roots which can reach down 40 feet into the soil in order to find water for its sustenance. Perhaps this is one reason why jojoba oil strengthens and improves the condition of the scalp and hair-shafts, whilst leaving a fine waxy sheen along the length of the hair.

The perfect combination of external nutrients for the scalp and hair are essential oils and jojoba. Essential oils, as we have seen elsewhere in this book, contribute greatly to the process of cell renewal, and most significantly, in increasing the resilience of the cell membrane so that it is not so easily broken down by other forces. I recommend jojoba as a base for all hair and scalp problems.

Treatment of hair problems

Dry, lacklustre hair

2 drops myrtle oil
2 drops lavender oil
3-4 teaspoons jojoba oil

Dandruff

4 drops tea tree oil
2 drops bergamot oil
3-4 teaspoons jojoba oil

Excess grease

2 drops orange oil
2 drops lemon oil
3-4 teaspoons jojoba oil

Hair loss

2 drops rosemary oil
2 drops geranium oil
3-4 teaspoons jojoba oil

Normal hair

1 drop orange oil
1 drop lavender oil
1 drop geranium oil
3-4 teaspoons jojoba oil

Choose one of the above blends, and apply to the scalp by sectioning the hair. When the scalp and hair roots are completely saturated, work the oil along the length of the hair right to the ends. Massage thoroughly for 5 minutes and then gather the hair into a scrunch band (if you have long hair) and wrap the hair in a clean, dry towel. If the weather is cold, a warmed towel feels luxuriously comforting. The towel's warmth encourages the essential oils to penetrate the skin and make their way into the dermis where they can work their magic. On a hot day you will not need the use of a warm towel as the air temperature, combined with the warmth of the head, will be sufficient heat.

Commercial hair conditioners can be applied and then rinsed off within minutes because they are non-organic substances (chemical polymers) which, like fabric conditioners, are positively charged and only give an illusion of healthy hair but without correcting the problem. (There are no positive charges in nature, only negative or negative/positive mixes.) Conditioning hair with aromatic hair treatment oils is completely different as they need to be in contact with the head for a minimum of 1-2 hours. If wished, the treatment oil can be left on the hair overnight, but this can be messy and you will almost certainly get oil on the pillowcase. Protect the pillow by placing a hand towel on top of the pillow, but inside the pillow case.

To remove treatment oil, use a mild shampoo (as natural as possible) and apply a little shampoo and water to make an emulsion. Massage the scalp for a minute or two before rinsing away. Then wash in the normal way. Dry hair feels silkier and softer; greasy hair, with time, will become normal; thin, fly-away hair becomes more luxuriant; and dandruff can be effectively banished.

Essential oil shampoo

For consistency of fragrance as well as action, buy an unperfumed shampoo (there are now several on the market) and add your own fragrance. According to your hair type, add one of the following essential oil combinations, or your own personal favourite:

- Lemon and bergamot
- Myrtle and lavender
- Tea tree and lemon
- Tea tree and bergamot
- Rosemary and geranium
- Lemon and geranium

The rough proportions should be 8-10 drops essential oil to every 100ml shampoo, so to a 250ml bottle of shampoo, add up to 25 drops of essential oil. Tilt bottle to side to mix.

Hair rinse

No hair rinse will effect a permanent cure, as the essences in water are very dilute and only poured through the hair, but regular use of an aromatic hair rinse will compound the benefits already obtained from an aromatic treatment oil. Rosemary or cypress will help to strengthen weak hair prone to falling out, by improving the circulation. Lemon and bergamot are particularly suitable for greasy hair and will impart a fresh, citrus smell, leaving the scalp tinglingly clean and invigorated. Myrtle oil, being hyperaemic, brings a rush of blood to the skin's surface, making it an ideal addition to the morning hair washing routine, leaving you energized and mentally alert. Moreover, the lingering fragrance of an aromatic hair rinse makes you feel special.

A hair rinse is very inexpensive and simple to make. To a 2 litre bottle of water add around 20 drops of essential oil. Shake vigorously before each use.

Head massage

Inside our head lies the control centre that governs our body, sending messages to the rest of our body to make it function, and empowering the brain to make rational decisions about health, happiness and life in general. Why then do we sometimes feel confused, heavy-headed, depressed or tense? Too much worry and anxiety can reduce the amount of blood flowing to the top of the head; too much stress makes the body produce more androgen which causes hair loss; too much tension in the head and shoulders interfers with the proper flow of lymph so it cannot perform its duties of bringing lymphocytes to the area and taking away waste matter. These reasons explain why we cannot function properly whilst under stress, and seek ways to disconnect ourselves from our 'dis-function'.

A head massage, whilst not a magic wand to relieve us of all problems, will certainly bring about a remarkable improvement in our well-being and mental clarity. Even if only carried out once a week, a head massage can:

• improve the flow of blood to the head
• help with elimination of toxins via lymph drainage
• release tension stored in muscle fibre of the scalp and neck
• help to lift the spirits by using euphoric essential oils.

Nothing could be simpler than a head massage, and it is not even necessary to apply fatty oils to the hair. Taking myrtle oil as an example, put a drop or two of essential oil onto the fingertips, spread evenly over the tips of thumbs and fingers and massage the scalp. Use slow, rhythmic movements if you are feeling tense or delicate. Use more robust, vigorous movements if you have been feeling lethargic and confused.

Begin with thumbs on the temples and fingers at the hairline and keeping thumbs still, move the scalp with your fingertips (see Figure 6). Massage the entire scalp (as if you were washing your hair), finishing at the nape of the neck, and then taking the back of the neck between thumb and fingers of one hand, gently squeeze the flesh so that the fingers and thumb slide across the skin and meet in the middle of the neck (see Figure 7). Locate tender areas along the neck and pinch flesh between fingers and thumb (do one side of the neck at a time). Let your fingers do the asking and find out where the sore spots are – be sensitive to your body and give it some TLC where it is crying out for

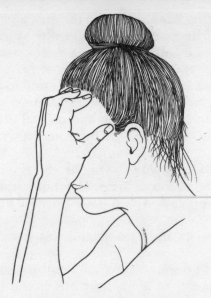

Figure 6. Massaging the head

attention. There is no set time to giving yourself a head massage – your arms will probably decide. After massaging the head, apply pressure to the nodes to encourage the flow of lymph (see Figure 8).

Whilst massaging your head and smoothing away the knots of tension, why not imagine you are massaging away the cause of your problem. If the cause of tension is your inability to speak up for yourself or to be assertive enough, talk to yourself for a few minutes and find out why you think you can't do something.

Essential oils are not magical potions which can transform a wish into a reality, but they can impart clarity of thought, a strength of purpose, peace and serenity.

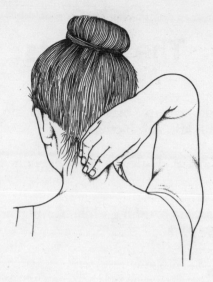

Figure 7. Massaging the nape of the neck

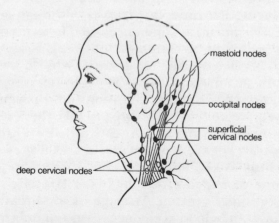

Figure 8. Lymph nodes of the head

Chapter 7

The breasts

The problems: Sagging breasts; breasts too large or too small; stretch marks and blemishes.

The causes: Loss of elasticity – gravity, genetics; rapid weight gain or loss.

The solutions: Skin brushing while bathing; aromatic baths; massage; chest pack.

The breasts

Breasts are the ultimate symbol of womanly beauty, proclaiming our ability to produce and feed babies, as well as being a much-vaunted sexual attractant. No more than a mass of adipose tissue until hormonally changed into a milk-producing machine, our breasts, although coveted objects of adornment, are often neglected in terms of physical care, merely to be crammed into bras, basques and 'bodies' – completely taken for granted. Why do we spend five minutes cleaning our teeth, 20 minutes having a face mask, another 10-15 minutes cleansing and massaging our face and yet give no time to the breasts. Like the rest of our body, the breasts contain connective tissue which can become disarranged, lymph vessels and nodes which syphon off toxins and infections, and muscle fibre, which can become damaged either by being stretched or by contracting under tension. Massage of the breasts with aromatic oils can help to keep our breasts not only in good shape but also in good health, too.

When weight has been gained or lost too rapidly, the skin sometimes scars, leaving a constant reminder of our weight change in the form of tiny silver lines. Stretch marks cannot vanish in two weeks as it takes far longer than that for new skin to grow, but it is possible to reduce the visible scarring over a period of time. Just by massaging the breasts with one of the aromatic blends, and by increasing the elasticity of the skin, the effect of stretch marks will lessen.

Nowhere on the female body is the saying 'beauty is more than skin deep' more pertinent. If we take care of the breasts, helping the lymphatic glands to rid the body of poisons, and applying the healing effects of essential oils when necessary, I believe we can help to prevent ill health.

Whatever the problem, the regime is the same.

Skin brushing in the bath

Spend at least one evening a week taking care of your breasts. Begin with a relaxing aromatic bath and whilst soaking in the healing fragrance, take a nail brush and, without using much pressure, run the bristles from the breast bone out to the armpit. Brush across the entire breast, always in the direction of the armpits where the axillary lymph nodes are housed. Lifting up one arm, brush the underside of the upper arm towards the armpit, and then brush the armpit itself. Underneath this area of skin, which has made billions of pounds for the deodorant industry, lies a cluster of lymph nodes, vitally placed to drain lymph from the arms and breasts (see Figure 9). If we could see the nodes and the myriad lymph vessels converging on them, it would look like a network of railway lines converging on a central station. And what do we do with this incredible mainline station? We shave off the hairs and slap anti-perspirant over every square millimetre of surface skin.

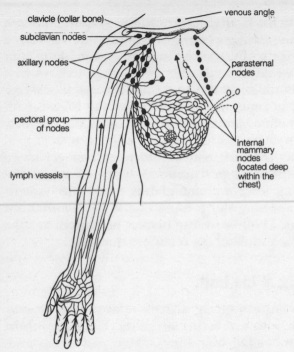

Figure 9. Lymph nodes of the breast

In order to facilitate the healthy flow of lymph and to remove any residues of anti-perspirant or deodorant, brush the armpit until it tingles – nothing too rough, just gentle stimulation, and understanding the importance of this area, give the body a well-deserved break from time to time and go without deodorant or anti-perspirant.

Breast massage

The massage techniques are the same for every woman, the only difference being the blend of oils used. If you are happy with the size of your breasts use **vetivert in camellia** blend. If you feel that your breasts are too small and would like to try to increase their size, use the **geranium blend**. Women who have large breasts and would like to reduce and tone them slightly, use the **rose in jojoba** blend. For recipes, see pages 21-22.

Whichever blend is chosen, and whether or not a change in size is achieved, massage will improve the muscle tone of the breasts, the feel of the skin will become silky smooth, and the general health of the breasts will be improved.

Massaging the breasts, of necessity, also massages many lymph nodes – those little drains which take away poisons and dead matter from the mammaries and, just as importantly, bring a fresh supply of lymph containing lymphocytes to recognize and kill unwanted organisms, such as bacteria and viruses. Each of us is home to a 'cocktail of germs' which, unless destroyed by our immune system, will be allowed to breed and eventually cause havoc with our health. So by massaging our breasts with a simple blend of essential oils and high quality fatty oils, we are promoting the flow of lymph as well as bringing the healing powers of essential oils to this part of our body.

The nightly massage routine

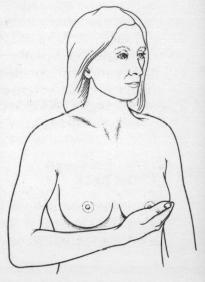

Every night I spend about five minutes working on my breasts, using either the **vetivert blend** or the **geranium blend**. Using your chosen blend, massage one breast at a time. With your right hand sweep your palm under your left breast and out to the armpit, repeating this movement several times (see Figure 10). Apply more oil whenever necessary and smooth into the breast, begin-

Figure 10. Massage of the breasts

ning in the centre of your chest (the sternum), bringing
your hand out to the edge of the breast, over the top of the
breast, and back to the sternum. Continue this circular
massage for a minute or two. Either side of the sternum,
located between the ribs, are the parasternal lymph nodes
which not only drain the mammaries but also receive lymph
from the liver, diaphragm, pericardium and intercostal
(between the ribs) spaces. Apply firm fingertip pressure to
these spots and if tender to the touch, these nodes are in
need of your attention. By keeping these nodes in good
health we not only aid the health of the breasts but improve
liver function and good metabolism.

Next, apply oil to the area under the collarbone (clavicle) and out to the edge of the chest. Using the tips of the
first three fingers, massage the muscles – 'nature's bra
straps' – which support the weight of the breast. By massaging these muscles we are performing two important functions – maintaining good muscle tone, and stimulating the
lymph nodes sited here (see Figure 9).

Change hands, and with the left hand repeat all movements on right breast.

The main thoracic duct runs up the back, in parallel with
the spine, and drains its lymph into the left venous angle
(see Figure 9). Lymph from the right side of the chest, face
and head drains into the right venous angle. These points
can be massaged at any time of day and should be included
as an integral part of breast care.

Effective though this massage is, it need take no longer
than the removal of make-up and cleaning of teeth.

Chest pack

Sometimes the skin in the centre of the chest (from just
above the cleavage to the base of the neck) becomes spotty,
which is the last thing we want to have when wearing a

low-cut dress for a special occasion. Just as a face pack instantly refreshes and revitalises the skin, so too does a chest pack.

Kaolin, water and myrtle mask

2 tablespoons kaolin
2 teaspoons water
2 drops myrtle oil

Mix the kaolin, water and myrtle oil together and spread across the chest. After applying the mask it is advisable to lie down for approximately 15 minutes whilst the clay is drying. As dry clay tends to flake off it is a good idea to cover the chest with a hand towel before walking to the bathroom and rinsing off the mask. Be assured that kaolin rinses easily out of the towels. Use either a hand-held shower spray or a large pad of cotton wool soaked in water. If using the latter, keep rinsing the cotton wool under a running tap until the last of the clay has been removed. Pat dry and apply a light coating of **rose in jojoba**.

Fuller's earth may be used instead of kaolin, but its darker colour can be a problem with light towelling.

Breast Care Plan													
Day	1	2	3	4	5	6	7	8	9	10	11	12	13	14
Bathe and skin brush	✓	✓	✓	✓	✓	✓	✓	✓	✓	✓	✓	✓	✓	✓
Massage	✓	✓	✓	✓	✓	✓	✓	✓	✓	✓	✓	✓	✓	✓
Chest pack			✓				✓					✓		

Chapter 8

The back
and shoulders

The problems: Congested skin dotted with pimples; greasy
skin with open pores; dull-looking skin; tension in back and
neck; stiffness in the shoulders.

The causes: Lack of movement (of skin and muscles); stagnation; lack of air; improper diet; dehydration.

The solutions: Bathing – use of friction with friction strip;
skin brushing; back compress (body wrap); aromatic back-
pack; massage.

A beautiful back

All of the above problems respond to bathing with aromatic
oils, friction and skin brushing. Some of them – congested
skin, greasy skin and dull-looking skin – can be treated by a
body wrap or back pack, both fun to experience. For stiffness and tension in the neck and shoulders, there are some
simple techniques to use yourself. If you have a partner or
friend to give you a full back massage, there are simple
instructions given for the second person to follow.

Anti-bacterial essential oils

The wonderful thing about using essential oils to treat a
spotty back is that bacteria do not become resistant to essential oils. There are many essential oils which will tackle the

problem of bacteria-induced spots and even if there was a chance that bacteria were becoming resistant to one particular oil, there are always many more to choose from.

All essential oils are anti-bacterial. Some are more powerful than others, while some work in lower concentrations, but all have the ability to cleanse and sterilize the skin when in contact with it, whether in the bath, a compress, massage oil or body wrap.

Aromatic bath for the shoulders

Revitalize tired skin on the shoulders by taking an aromatic bath fragranced with one of the cleansing essential oils – myrtle, lavender, lemon, bergamot – and immerse your body right up to your neck in the aromatic water. The water should not be too hot, or too much blood will rush to your head causing a flushed look or even dizzyness. The ideal temperature is just above body temperature, at around 100°F(37°C). Depending on time constraints, relax and use the time for positive, empowering thoughts.

Congested skin on the back can be stimulated and improved by taking an aromatic bath with 6-10 drops of either myrtle, lavender, bergamot, geranium, rosemary or niaouli. Alternatively make your own blend such as 3 drops myrtle, 2 drops bergamot, 5 drops lavender. Agitate the water before stepping into the bath.

If your skin is greasy choose from lemon, patchouli, lavender, bergamot, niaouli, orange, rosemary, geranium or juniper.

If your skin is dry choose from sandalwood, rose, lavender, geranium or frankincense.

Skin brushing in the bath

Sit up in the bath and, taking the nail brush in your right

hand, run the bristles along your upper left arm from elbow
to shoulder and then from the crease of elbow to the armpit,
until the entire skin surface has been covered. Next, reach
your right arm across your left shoulder and brush across the
shoulders, and then brush from behind the neck to the
collarbone. Under the collarbone is a collection of lymph
nodes known as subclavian nodes which drain impurities
away from the upper chest and neck. Stimulating the skin in
this area will assist your body in its efforts to eliminate
unwanted matter. Women who wear bras with shoulder straps
are particularly vulnerable to congestion around the shoulders because for 8, 10, 16 hours a day there may be pressure
on the shoulders, and any pressure, no matter how slight, if
endured for protracted periods of time, will have a negative
effect. I don't like bras and whenever possible prefer to go
bra-less , and when I need to wear a bra it has to be strapless.

One more area which I believe is necessary to be brushed
is the armpit. The armpits house a mass of lymph nodes
clustered together, with lymph vessels radiating out from
them, like rays of the sun. These nodes are known as the
axillary lymph nodes and are vitally important in protecting
the health of the body and, in particular, the upper body,
chest and arms. Many of the most important lymph nodes
of the body are situated in areas where they are not vulnerable to injury. Like a hedgehog protecting his delicate belly
by curling into a ball, our lymph nodes are sited behind the
knees, in the crease of the elbow, in the armpits and in the
groin, so that if we curl up in the foetal position, the lymph
nodes are all protected. However they are also positioned
where they can be easily reached.

Friction rub in the bath

Because the surface area of the back is so great (about 18
per cent of our total skin surface), it is an ideal site for the

elimination of the body's toxins and waste products. If, for
example, we have been tempted to eat an entire box of
chocolates, it is very likely that within a day or two spots will
have broken out on the skin of the back. A spotty back can
also be caused by a build-up of sweat and sebum because it
is not being thoroughly cleansed. How wonderful it would
be if each one of us had a loving partner on hand to scrub
our back clean at every bath-time. Failing this, we can efficiently scrub away at the skin of our back by using a friction strip. There are a variety available in chemists and
department stores – sisal, pot-scourer-type, or towelling.

A towelling friction strip is quite easy to make for yourself
if it is not possible to purchase one. The length of a hand
towel is about right, from which you cut a 16cm wide strip.
For each handle use either 20cm pyjama cord or ribbon.
Tie a firm knot in the ribbon or cord and place the knotted
section on the end of towelling strip. Fold material over the
string and sew with strong thread.

Allow yourself to soak for at least ten minutes whilst
savouring the health-giving, aromatic vapours. Taking the
handles of the friction strip, draw it back and forth across
your back, until the skin tingles. When every square centimetre of skin has been covered, again immerse your body in
the fragrant waters for 5-10 minutes. Wash and dry as usual,
making sure that no residues of soap are left on the back.

Body wrap

A body wrap is the simplest and most effective way of
decongesting the skin of the back and shoulders , especially if you are not able to have a massage from someone
using essential oils. A body wrap can easily be carried out at
home on your own, but needs to be carefully planned in
advance. A body wrap or wet pack, as naturopaths call it, is
an effective way of drawing toxins from the body. The skin,

as the largest organ of the human body, is an important means of elimination.

Place a blanket on the bed, a sheet of plastic on top (an opened out black bin liner is ideal) and then a large bath towel. If you are alone it may be prudent to take the phone off the hook or switch on the answerphone as about one hour is needed for a body wrap to work effectively and you will be fairly immobile. A comfortably warm room is advisable. A body wrap is an excellent opportunity for taking a cat-nap, but if you find it difficult to drift off during the day, you could read a paperback book (nothing too heavyweight as you will be lying on your back holding the book above your face), switch on the radio or have your favourite music tapes playing in the background. Have a glass of water within reach, tissues and anything else you may want within the next hour.

A suitable compress can be made from an old cotton sheet (single size) folded or cut smaller, or from an old cotton pillowcase, cut down one side and end. Polyester/ cotton mixture is not suitable as polyester is non-absorbent. Remove all your clothes except perhaps your knickers and put on a towelling robe if you have one. Half-fill a hand basin with comfortably hot water and then add 6 drops of your chosen essential oil or combination of essential oils. The choice rests with you, but strongly recommended oils are bergamot, myrtle or lavender. A good combination is three drops each of either bergamot and lavender or myrtle and lavender.

Agitate the water to ensure that oils are fully dispersed and dip in the cotton material. Wring out excess water and immediately place into a plastic bag to conserve the heat (a carrier bag is fine). In your bedroom, take off the robe, place the compress in the centre of the bath towel and lie down on your back, positioning yourself so that the compress comes into contact with your back. Fold the edges of the bath towel over your front so that only your arms, legs and head are exposed. Flick the blanket over your legs and abdomen leaving your arms out if you wish to read or snuggle inside if you wish to sleep. By now you will be looking like a sausage roll, but what a treat for your back!

Naturopathic practioners, such as the late Harry Benjamin, have been advocating wet packs since the early part of the twentieth century and firmly believe that many diseases are attributable to a malfunction of the skin. The body wrap allows us to draw impurities out of the body in a simple, relaxed way. This type of compress is one of the treatments given in some health spas. Allowing the client to sleep whilst wrapped in fluffy towels and with gentle music in the background, contributes greatly to the overall feeling of well-being derived from spending time in a health spa – and it is this feeling of luxury and unhurriedness which, in part, commands the high price of such a spa.

Aromatic back pack

To refine skin of the upper back, especially between the shoulder blades where sebum can clog pores and spots accumulate, treat your skin to a back pack with a difference. It's quite a messy operation and must be planned in advance. As the mask has to be in place for at least half an hour, choose some music to listen to or switch on the radio. Place a plastic sheet on the bed with a bath towel on top. A plastic dustbin liner is ideal – just cut in half across its length and you have enough for two back packs.

Myrtle is particularly good for clearing spotty and congested skin, and is one of my favourite essential oils, being antiseptic and cleansing whilst having the most wonderful aroma, but any one of the following oils would be effective: bergamot, lemon, orange, lavender, tea tree, niaouli, rose or geranium.

100g fuller's earth powder
sufficient water to mix to a firm paste
5-6 drops myrtle oil
Mix ingredients together.

Spread the clay thickly over the towel – an area large enough to cover your back – and lie down carefully. The pack will feel cold to your skin at first, but soon warms up and by the end of half an hour it is very warm. Bring the loose ends of the towel over your front so that you are completely wrapped up with just your arms and legs exposed. If you are completely undressed you may want to cover your legs with another towel or blanket.

An aromatic back pack needs to be showered off and a hand-held shower attachment is ideal. Holding the towel tightly to your body, so that no clay drops onto the floor, make your way to the bathroom and step into the bath or shower before removing the towel.

The easiest way to deal with the clay adhering to the towel is to allow it to dry and then shake the towel in the garden. If you don't have a garden, shake the towel into the bath and then scoop out the clay and dispose of in a bin. To wash this much clay down the bath plughole requires gallons of water so, for the sake of conserving water, it is preferable and easier to dispose of the dried clay.

A messy task admittedly, but well worth the trouble if your back is greasy or dotted with pimples. The result is a tinglingly clean and clear skin.

Massage of the back and shoulders

If you have a partner willing and able to give you a back massage or you can persuade a friend, sister or partner to massage your back you will be able to experience the benefits of a back massage. So much tension can be soothed away with a few simple techniques and a simple blend of essential and fatty oils.

15ml (approximately 3 teaspoons) camellia, sweet almond oil or your choice of fatty oil
6-9 drops of your chosen oil, for example:

Relaxing blend

15ml camellia
3 drops sandalwood
2-3 drops lavender
3-4 drops patchouli

Invigorating blend

15ml camellia
2-3 drops myrtle
2 drops bergamot
3-4 drops lemon

Pour the oils into a bowl and mix with fingertips before beginning the massage.

A simple back massage

For a back massage to be truly effective, at least twenty minutes will be needed, and in this time the body can begin to feel cold, so make sure that the room is warm enough, and have the legs covered with a towel whilst the back is being worked on. You (or your friend) should be lying comfortably on a soft but firm surface, with a small cushion or pillow under the tummy or ankles (whatever makes you feel comfortable), and the masseur should kneel, sit or stand to one side at the level of recipient's hips. It is advisable to remove rings and watches, so they do not interfere with the massage.

The massage consists mainly of effleurage with some kneading of the areas of tension. Whoever is giving the massage should cover the palms of their hands with massage oil and stroke onto the back of the recipient until the entire skin surface is covered, then with hands flat on the back at hip level (see Figure 11), slide them up the spine to the

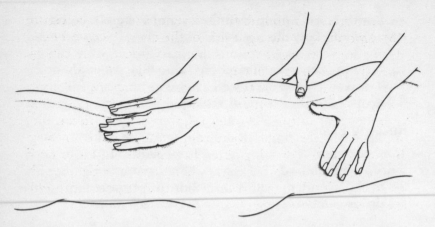

Figure 11. Massaging the back   **Figure 12.** Massaging the sore spots

base of the neck, using firm pressure. Draw hands out to the shoulders, and slide them back down to where you started but with a lighter pressure. Vary the pressure and ask the recipient to tell you if there are any sore areas. Using the pads of the thumbs, locate the sore spots and press and rub the skin in a circular movement until the soreness eases a little (see Figure 12). Add more oil whenever necessary and continue to effleurage the back. Then massage the shoulders using the thumbs and fingers to smoothe and knead the skin, as the shoulders hold a lot of tension. Finish with more effleurage and then, using tissues or paper kitchen towel, blot off the excess oil.

After the back massage, it is advisable to massage the points on the chest just above and below the clavicle as this is where lymph drains into the bloodstream. Nature really is incredible – she has positioned the main lymph drains on the front of the body where they can be reached even if we do not have a partner to massage our back. The main thoracic duct runs up the back, in parallel with the spine, and drains its lymph into the left venous angle (see Figure 13). Lymph from the right side of the chest, face and head drains into the right venous angle. These points can be massaged at any time of day.

If you do not have access to a massage, you can still apply some aromatic oil to your shoulders and neck where tension is stored and stiffness is often registered. Remember, too, that many lymph nodes drain from this area and by massaging, stroking and pressing different points around your neck shoulders and upper back, you will help your body not only to feel better in the short term but to function more efficiently in the long term.

Back and Shoulders Plan

Day	1	2	3	4	5	6	7	8	9	10	11	12	13	14
Bathe and skin brush	✓	✓	✓	✓	✓	✓	✓	✓	✓	✓	✓	✓	✓	✓
Friction of back	✓		✓		✓		✓		✓		✓		✓	
Aromatic back pack				✓				✓				✓		
Body wrap							✓							✓
Self-massage of neck and shoulders	✓					✓					✓			

Chapter 9

Tummy, waist and abdomen

The problems: Excess fat; wrinkles; tension stored in the solar plexus.

The causes: Fat deposits; toxic wastes; stress.

The solutions: Aromatic baths; skin brushing; massage; cling-film wrap.

Tummy and waist

The tummy is often the first place where we notice an increase in weight, or rather an increase in girth. When skirts no longer fit and trousers will not zip up, we know that we have amassed excess fat. But why does fat accumulate so easily around the waist?

One reason may be that there are no lymph nodes on the front of the torso. From the navel upwards, the lymph vessels take fluids and drain them to the axillary glands under the arms, and from the navel downwards, the lymph drains to the inguinal nodes in the groin (see Figure 13). Because there are no lymph nodes actually at the waist, it is easy for cells to become crammed full of fat. By encouraging the flow of lymph to the nodes which will filter and break down the fat deposits, we can help control the size of our waists. From the inguinal nodes lymph flows to the intestinal and lumbar trunks (which also drain fluid from the entire abdominal cavity) into the cisterna chyli, which

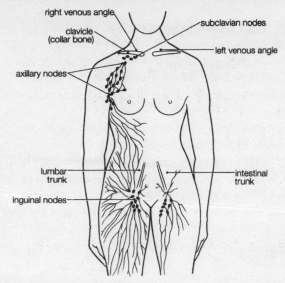

Figure 13. Lymph nodes of the tummy, waist and abdomen

lies deep in the body, next to the vertebrae.

From the cisterna chyli, which is on a level with the navel, but deeper in the body, the lymph flows into the thoracic duct and travels up the body almost parallel with the spine before dividing into two parts at the level of the heart. The left fork drains into the left venous angle, a large vein sited above the left collar bone. Also draining into this vein is lymph from the left side of the face, head, chest and arm. Lymph from the right side of the head, face, chest and arm drains into the right lymphatic duct at the right venous angle above the right collar bone.

Aromatic baths

Bathe with oils such as juniper or orange which aid in the dispersal of unwanted fats and fluids, or bathe in essences which are hyperaemic (such as myrtle) and bring fresh blood to the skin's surface. This helps to tone and firm the tummy as fresh blood brings with it nutrients to feed the skin. Lymphatics are also stimulated, allowing fats to be broken down and carried away from the site, eventually to be expelled from the body. Many fats are recycled by the body simply because the liver is not able to cope with large quantities.

Stress release is of great importance when we are endeavouring to get rid of unwanted layers of fat. Stress affects people in different ways, and for some people too much stress can interfere with the efficient metabolism of the body allowing a build up of fatty deposits, so it is useful to add anti-stress oils to the bath, such as geranium, lavender and rose.

Skin brushing

Skin brushing of the abdomen is very effective because the concentration of adipose fat makes it difficult for essential oils to penetrate. Skin brushing stimulates the movement of fat and lymph and encourages drainage of unwanted toxins as well as the increased absorption of essential oils. If you intend to massage the tummy and waist later, skin brush the whole of the abdomen – the abdomen is the area from the diaphragm to the floor of the pelvis – as it will prepare the skin for the essential oil blends.

Taking the nail brush, stroke from the navel downwards to the 'knicker line', brushing the skin across the inguinal nodes at the top of the legs. Then brush from the navel upwards to the diaphragm, and skirting around the breasts, sweep up to the axillary nodes at the armpit.

Massage of tummy and waist

Massage of the tummy and waist can help to eliminate toxins, break up fatty deposits and encourage their dispersal, toning up the skin and underlying muscle so that wrinkles are reduced. If the flesh hurts when pinched between thumb and fingers, this could indicate that the tissues are home to stagnant wastes so choose the **lemongrass blend**. Choose the **juniper blend** if you are prone to occasional water retention and the unwanted inches around your waist contain not only fatty tissue but also excess fluid.

Apply the chosen oil blend to your skin and whilst lying down comfortably, take a handful of flesh from your lower abdomen and roll the fat between your fingers and thumbs, gently massaging the flesh towards you. Continue to do this over the whole of the tummy area, remembering to apply more oil blend whenever the skin loses its 'slip' and your skin has absorbed the massage oil. After 15 minutes, or when you feel that you have worked long enough, sweep your palm from the navel down to the 'knicker line' and from the navel up to the armpits so that the lymph nodes are encouraged to break down the fats and toxins and the lymphatic system can carry off the unwanted debris.

Cling-film wrap

An effective, though not permanent, way to whittle away the waist is to give yourself a cling-film wrap. The tummy and waist have so many fat cells clustered together that it is more difficult for essential oils to penetrate here. A cling-film wrap will aid the penetration of essential oils as well as encourage the elimination of water by causing the skin to sweat.

A cling-film wrap can be left in place for one or two hours, but for best results leave on overnight, perhaps prior to a special occasion, when you want to squeeze into a figure-hugging item of clothing.

Firstly, massage the waist with a blend of essential oils, such as the **lemongrass blend** or the **juniper blend** and then wrap a sizeable length of cling-film around the waist and tummy. If left on overnight the essential oils will be unable to evaporate and will be forced into the skin. The skin will also sweat because of the close proximity of the plastic. After use, the cling-film should be cut off and discarded. This is not a permanent way to banish fat from the tummy and waist, but ideal for an instant tone-up and is a technique used in many beauty salons.

The solar plexus

The solar plexus is sited halfway between the navel and the end of the breastbone, and is a very sensitive area. If we are under stress or have experienced something traumatic (even watching the news on television) we may find that the area of the solar plexus is sore to touch. You may also find that just under the surface of the skin this part of your abdomen feels tight and hard, as though the muscles have become 'knotted up'. This is precisely what has happened but tension in the solar plexus can very easily be massaged away.

Solar plexus massage

Apply a little massage oil, such as **rose in camellia**, to the area between the navel and the sternum (see Figure 14). Lie on the bed and rest your hand over the solar plexus and just breathe peacefully for a few minutes. Be aware of the tension under your hand. Can you feel a tightness? Is the underlying flesh hard to the touch?

Using both hands, place fingertips on the solar plexus, so the backs of the fingers are touching each other. Take a deep breath and as you breathe out, gently press the finger-tips into the tender area. As you breathe in, allow the fingers to rise up as the diaphragm expands, and again gently press the fingertips into the solar plexus with the out breath. (This is difficult to do if the fingernails are very long.) Continue in this manner until the solar plexus has lost its

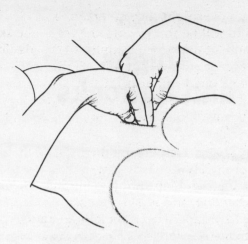

Figure 14. Massaging the solar plexus

tenderness, but at the most for 5-10 minutes. Finally, apply a little more **rose in camellia** and gently rub the abdomen, sweeping your hand in a clockwise circle. Rest for a few minutes, or make this the last thing you do before going to sleep, to ensure a restful night.

Tummy, Waist and Abdomen Plan														
Day	1	2	3	4	5	6	7	8	9	10	11	12	13	14
Bathe and skin brush	✓	✓	✓	✓	✓	✓	✓	✓	✓	✓	✓	✓	✓	✓
Massage of tummy	✓		✓		✓		✓		✓		✓			
Cling-film wrap				✓			✓				✓			
Solar plexus massage		✓				✓				✓				✓

Chapter 10

Thighs and buttocks

The problems: Thighs: cellulite; fat thighs; dull, lifeless skin; excess fat (poor metabolism).
Buttocks: dull lifeless skin; pimples; buttock 'droop'; fat; stretch marks.

The causes: Toxins in tissues; poor metabolism; stagnation – poor circulation; lack of exercise; insufficient nutrition – inside and out.

The solutions: Aromatic bathing; skin brushing; massage; moisturizing and nourishing the skin.

Cellulite

If you have areas of cellulite on your thighs you are not alone, as cellulite affects almost 80 per cent of Western women at some stage of their lives. The good news is that cellulite is not permanent. Even though cellulite rarely responds to dieting and does not always respond to exercise, it does respond, fairly rapidly, to massage with specific essential oils.

Cellulite is not a true disease, in the sense of an irreversible pathological change, but a visual warning that the body is not functioning properly. (It should not be confused with cellulitis, which is a medical condition.) In fact, the lumpy thighs and less-than-beautiful buttocks are trying to tell you that the body is slowly being poisoned. Toxins are not being flushed away, but stored in the fat cells of the thighs, buttocks and upper arms. Why are these areas chosen as dumping grounds for the body? It is because the body sends all of the excess toxins that it cannot manage to eliminate through the lymph, blood stream, liver and kidneys, and normal elimination processes, into the extemities of the body – away from the vital organs needed to support life. In short, the thighs, buttocks and upper arms are used as a rubbish dump. The fat cells in these areas, when invaded by toxins which should have been evacuated from the body via the normal channels of elimination (excretion, urination and perspiration), become sponge-like and absorb fluid. Toxins are not only created by eating cream cakes and drinking vast quantities of alcohol, but are also products of metabolism – the debris left after the body cells have repaired themselves, and can be the result of eating large quantities of protein, for example when living on a diet of fast-food hamburgers.

Another contributing factor to the development of cellulite is any form of chronic stress, resulting in nervous anxiety. When the body is suffering severe stress it does not function efficiently and, especially when we 'eat for comfort', the excess toxins that the body cannot deal with end up on the thighs and upper arms.

Cellulite is the term used to describe the pitted appearance of the skin when it is pinched between the fingers – orange peel is an accurate description of the problem, and in France it is known as *'peau d'orange'*. The nickname of *'culotte de cheval'* has also been given to the condition, as cellulite is most often found on the outside of the thighs, which can give our legs the appearance of wearing jodhpurs. The sense of touch can also detect the presence of cellulite as the skin can be very tender to the touch, and if squeezed, very painful.

The skin is a mirror of internal health, and often when

the correct oil is chosen, both the internal problem and the skin condition will be improved as many skin problems have aromatic solutions. Congestion of the skin is often symptomatic of a poor circulation, as it is the circulating blood which brings a supply of oxygen to the skin cells and keeps them functioning healthily.

When the skin is congested the first step on the road to recovery is an aromatic bath, as essential oils have the ability to decongest tissues and help the body to eliminate toxins. Essence of lavender and rose are very powerful antiseptic agents but at the same time act gently on the skin, and can therefore be used for baths and massage. Cellulite is a visible sign of congestion, not only of the skin, but of the organs of elimination. A **lemongrass blend** or **juniper blend**, when used in massage of the affected areas, has a draining effect and stimulates the flow of lymph. Cellulite has probably accrued over a long period of time and cannot possibly be banished by a quick 15-minute massage, no matter what essential oils are used. Patience and effort are required if you wish to see an improvement in the appearance and texture of the thighs.

In order to create an optimum situation for eliminating toxins, fats and excess water from the thighs and buttocks, the thighs must be skin brushed thoroughly, taking care also to brush the 'knicker line' – the area of the body where the inguinal nodes are to be found. Stimulation of this area, followed by massage with specific essential and fatty oils, is a most effective way to banish cellulite from the thighs.

Obesity

Obesity is the result of eating far more calories than our body can burn up through daily activity, and instead of being used as fuel for energy, the fat cells become full – rather like a greedy hamster's storecupboard, where the pile of food is never used up, but continues to grow – and the bulkier we become. The problem is exacerbated when we eat large quantities of fats, especially saturated fats such as cream, butter and fatty meats, because the body simply cannot eliminate the excess, and therefore it becomes part of us. The saying 'you are what you eat' is unfortunately very true.

Sitting for long periods every day and sedentary work are major factors in loss of muscle tone in the buttocks. Toxins and fats are squashed by the weight of the body pressing down on a relatively small area – the buttocks. The upper thighs also suffer from prolonged periods of sitting, especially the back of the thighs where the circulation can be seriously impaired by pressure from the edge of a chair.

Obesity, lack of muscle tone and stubborn areas of fat will respond to physical massage, especially when used with essential oils that have a stimulating effect on metabolism, such as grapefruit oil for the gall bladder, juniper for the kidneys, lemon and orange for the liver. A **lemongrass blend** or a **juniper blend** used in regular massage of the thighs and buttocks has a very toning and slimming effect.

Stretch marks

Stretch marks often accompany cellulite or excess fat in the thighs. If the living skin is considerably overstretched by rapid weight gain or loss, ruptures can occur in the structure of the corium which become visible as pale stripes, so-called 'distension striae', commonly known as 'stretch marks'.

The corium is a dense network of collagen fibres intermingled with elastic fibres which allows the skin to stretch and return to normal. The cells which originate in the basal layer of the epidermis undergo step-by-step transformation, leading to the migration of cells from the basement layer to the surface, a process which takes about 30 days. This means that by applying essential and fatty oils in generous amounts, over a period of time we will be able to influence the new growth of cells which will replace the ruptured skin tissue, and the stretch marks will eventually disappear.

With all problems of the thighs, massage with **lemongrass blend** or **juniper blend** can be very successful. Once you've tackled the cellulite and reduced the excess fat, massage with **vetivert in camellia** helps the stretch marks to recede and become less visible.

Aromatic bathing

Take a morning bath if this is your chosen time of day to spend on yourself, perhaps getting up an hour earlier than normal if you have a busy day ahead. The morning is an ideal time of day to tackle cellulite and excess fat of thighs and buttocks, since the very nature of the massage, the pre-massage skin brushing and the choice of essential oils are all fairly stimulating, and if used late at night, may interfere with your ability to fall asleep.

Add to the bath those essential oils which are refreshing and uplifting. The zest of oranges is a natural choice to revitalize and set the mood for positive action. To this you could add a few drops of clary sage if your emotions need a 'lift'. It's especially good for Monday morning lethargy, when the prospect of going to work brings a feeling of depression and inertia and all you want to do is crawl back into bed.

Although some essential oils have specific effects on the body – such as the diuretic properties of juniper oil – it is not necessary to use these oils in the bath if you will be applying liberal quantities of these essential oils in massage. Just choose an oil or oils which will refresh and cleanse the skin in preparation for a massage. Ideal candidates would be rose, bergamot, geranium or rosemary.

Skin brushing

After relaxing for a few minutes in a fresh, uplifting fragrance, use a nailbrush to stimulate the skin with firm pressure strokes, upward from knee to thigh until all the thigh has been covered with brush strokes. Your skin will feel tingly and may even turn reddish, but this is a temporary effect, caused by a rush of blood to the surface of the skin, and is of great benefit. Position yourself so that you have access to every part of your thighs, if necessary lifting your legs clear of the water in order to brush the backs of the thighs.

Now brush one buttock at a time, shifting your weight so that you have complete access to one side of your body. Stroke the bristles of the nailbrush from the buttock crease, out to the hipbone and continue round to the pelvic area and brush round the 'knicker line', ending at the inguinal nodes in the groin (see Figure 15). Continue to brush the skin of the buttock until it has been completely covered and the entire skin surface tingles pleasantly. Then change your position and do the same on the other side of your body.

Relax in the water for as long as you feel comfortable or have time, allowing the essential oils in the water to penetrate into the skin.

Massage of the thighs

Massage of the thighs can be carried out whilst standing but I find it easiest to massage my thighs whilst lying on top of my bed. Either a sofa or a bed could be used but do protect the furniture first with an old sheet. After your morning/ evening bath (whichever time of day is convenient) you need to spend 15-30 minutes on each leg. Get everything to hand that you will need, such as the massage blend, a glass of water, tissues, etc, and don't forget to switch on the answerphone or take the phone off the hook. An hour can seem like a long time when there is no visual or auditory stimulation, so why not use the time to brush up on a foreign language by listening to a language tape, or play a favourite piece of music. If you are a television fiend like me, why not combine an evening of massage with your favourite programmes.

Before you begin, take a critical look at yourself in a full-length mirror. Note the shape and size of your thighs. Lock that sight into your memory , because each day as you look at yourself in the mirror you will see a gradual transformation. Not only will the shape of the thighs improve but also the appearance of the skin will be smoother and more refined, and the texture of the skin will improve, so that your fingers as well as your eyes will know that the special oil blends and massage techniques are working.

Take the massage oil of your choice – **juniper blend**, **lemongrass blend**, **vetivert in camellia** or jojoba in camellia. Position yourself comfortably – you may wish to sit up in order to massage your thighs, or you may wish to lean on one side on one elbow and massage your thigh with the other hand (see Figure 16).

Apply the chosen oil, a little at a time, to one thigh, noting how it seeps into the skin. Beginning just above the knee work the oil into the skin in small patches, and continue to build up further areas of oiled skin until the entire thigh has been covered. Reposition your leg as necessary, to gain access to every part of the thigh.

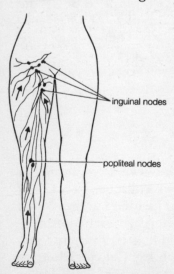

inguinal nodes

popliteal nodes

Figure 15. Lymph nodes of the legs

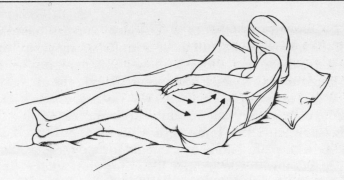

Figure 16. Massaging the thighs

Using fingertip pressure, stroke the fingers up the leg – not too forcefully and yet not too gently. You will be able to feel areas of discomfort, nobbles of fat under the skin, or crystals of salt, etc. Continue to apply more of the massage oil blend, working it into any 'problem areas' (see figure 17). Be sensitive to your body, spending more time massaging sore spots, before sweeping the palm of the hand up the thigh to the top of the leg, and ending by stroking the fingers around the 'knicker line'. Apply massage oil to the inguinal nodes and massage for a few minutes (see Figure 15). At first this area

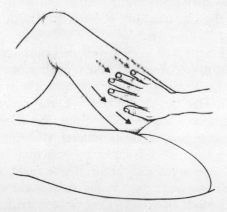

Figure 17. Massaging the inner thighs

may feel sensitive and tender to the touch. The first blend to use is the **lemongrass blend** as we want to 'spring clean' the connective tissue and allow the powerful lemongrass oil to 'burn up' the toxins which have accumulated over the years. The added essences of citrus oils will cleanse, detoxify and help the body's lymphatic system to drain more easily.

Massage with the **lemongrass blend** is followed by massage with plain jojoba or camellia for a day or two and then massage with the **juniper blend** for another few days and then back to jojoba or camellia. Depending on your results, you can then choose to go back to the **lemongrass blend** for further work on the underlying tissues, or if you are happy with the new shape of your thighs, use the **vetivert in camellia blend** to plump up the tissues and add a more youthful appearance.

Massage of the buttocks

If your buttocks have lost their youthful curves, and the cheeks no longer have firm definition but droop and merge ingloriously into the back of the thighs, then this area deserves a lot of attention. It is possible to rejuvenate the buttocks and bring back a firm contour, but only by consistent effort of working on this area with the massage oil blends.

The fingertips are very small in comparison to your buttocks, and therefore it will take considerable time for you to complete the massage of just one buttock, probably about half an hour. The larger the buttock, the more time it will take, or, if time is a scarce commodity, the thoroughness of the massage may have to be sacrificed. When you first begin this intensive form of self-massage, you may feel tired and your fingers and arms may ache. If you really feel that it is too much to cope with, then build up gradually – doing 5-15 minutes on each buttock, take a rest and then spend another 5-15 minutes on each buttock. At the end of each

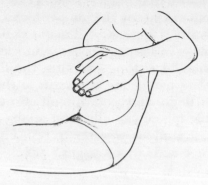

Figure 18. Massaging the buttocks

buttock-massage, sweep your hands round to the 'knicker-line' and then, with your hand between your legs, sweep from the buttock region round to the inguinal nodes in your groin. As lemongrass and citrus essential oils can be irritating to mucus membranes, ensure that the oils do not come into contact with the vagina, as they could cause irritation.

Using either the **lemongrass blend** or the **juniper blend** of oils, massage oil into one buttock, applying more oil as it is absorbed by the skin. I find that the best way to massage the buttocks is to be semi-reclining. Lie on top of your bed, on your side, with buttock to be worked on uppermost, and leg bent (see Figure 18).

Use fingertip massage to work the oil blend into the entire skin surface, paying particular attention to the area where buttock meets thigh. Use firm strokes here, and work on any portion of skin that feels knotty or lumpy under the surface. Press and probe the flesh in this area, which has been squashed and flattened for so many years of being sat on. Even after only a few evenings' massage of this area, a difference can be seen in the shape and definition of the cheeks, and if the buttocks are massaged regularly, it is possible to regain a youthful contour to the buttocks.

As an alternative to using the **lemongrass blend** you can massage the buttocks using the **juniper blend**, which will be especially effective if there is any fluid retention.

The final stage in massage of the buttocks is the use of **vetivert in camellia** to tone and firm the flesh. Massage everyday, paying particular attention to the area where buttock meets thigh, and work the oil into the skin. With the remarkable oils of camellia and jojoba blended with essential oils, it really is possible to rejuvenate the body. Recipes for the blends are on pages 21-22.

Shiatsu channels

I find it interesting to know which shiatsu meridians I am working on when I massage my thighs and buttocks, and include the following information for anyone else who is fascinated by the wisdom of shiatsu.

All shiatsu channels cross the thighs and buttocks. They are: bladder, gall bladder, spleen, liver, stomach, kidney, triple heater, small intestine, large intestine, lung, heart and heart constrictor.

'Meridian shiatsu' is a developemnt of 'Zen shiatsu', which places the emphasis on working along the channels of energy rather than treating specific points located along the channels. For example, the gall bladder channel located on the outside of each leg, runs all the way up the outside of the leg to the thighs and buttocks (and then upwards across the torso ending on the side of the head above the ear). When this channel is massaged with the **lemongrass blend** or **juniper blend** of oils, there will be an improvement in the condition of the gall bladder which is responsible for storing bile produced by the liver. It is the bile acids from the gall bladder that emulsify fats in the intestines and when this process becomes less than efficient, fat cannot be broken down properly and begins to build up in the body.

Another very important shiatsu channel is the stomach channel located on the front of the thighs, very close to the inguinal lymph nodes. Massage of this channel will aid the stomach in its important role of digestion and assimilation of nutrients. The stomach channel runs from the toes to the eye area.

Massage of the thighs will not only remove unwanted fat and toxins from the immediate area, but by toning and improving the body's vital organs, can assist the body in its essential function of metabolism.

Thighs and Buttocks Plan

Day	1	2	3	4	5	6	7	8	9	10	11	12	13	14
Bath and skin brush	✓	✓	✓	✓	✓	✓	✓	✓	✓	✓	✓	✓	✓	✓
Massage with lemongrass blend	✓	✓	✓											
Massage with juniper blend					✓	✓	✓							
Massage with jojoba or camellia				✓				✓	✓	✓			✓	✓
Massage with vetivert in camellia											✓	✓		

Chapter 11

Upper arms, elbows and neck

The problems: Flabby upper arms; cellulite; obesity; wrinkled elbows; lines on neck; rough or dead skin on elbows; dehydrated skin.

The causes: Loss of muscle tone; toxins; poor metabolism; age; pressure of leaning (elbows).

The solutions: Bathing; skin brushing; massage; astringent mask; moisturizing.

Aromatic baths

Bathing in aromatic water is beneficial for all problems relating to the upper arms, elbows and neck. Only a few drops of essential oil to a full tub of water are needed to create a therapeutic bath which will cleanse the skin, relax tense muscles, and open up the pores of the skin in readiness to receive massage oils. Many essential oils are excellent for the skin but especially recomended for their therapeutic properties and their fragrance are orange, myrtle, lemon, bergamot, lavender and rosemary.

Skin brushing

Skin brushing releases toxins from the body by the gentle stimulation of the skin's surface, and when incorporated into the aromatic bathing ritual, transforms the process of taking a bath into an important beauty treatment.

Take a nail brush and brush from wrist to elbow, gently at first, as many times as it takes to cover all of the forearm. Then repeat, using firmer pressure. Gently brush the folds of the elbow, where the cubital nodes are housed. These lymph glands are the first line of defence in detoxifying our hands, nails and forearms, and can become swollen and painful if we have a problem such as a septic finger. Now sweep from the bend of the elbow up to the top of the arm, if necessary lifting up your arm so that you can brush the underside. Continue the gentle brushing by sweeping the armpit, so that the axillary nodes are encouraged to work efficiently in carrying away the waste material dislodged by massage. Finally, sweep across the top of your shoulder, from the base of your neck out to tip of the shoulder, and bring the brush round to finish where the arm meets the body. Relax in the aromatic water for five minutes or so. Repeat on other arm.

The neck can also be skin brushed in the bath, with the brush stroking downwards from under the chin to the base of the neck. Work your way around the neck until all the skin, even the back of the neck, has been brushed. Next, sweep the brush from the back of the neck round to the front, finishing where the two ends of the clavicle meet. Using slightly firmer strokes, brush from the shoulder across the front of the chest, under the clavicle, and end at the top of the sternum. Repeat on the other side of the body.

Upper arms

Cellulite on upper arms

Cellulite on the upper arms is your body's 'overflow' tip where it has dumped toxins that it cannot deal with in other ways. Essential oils such as the **lemongrass blend**, which also contains orange and grapefruit, will remove toxins from the connective tissue, deep cleanse and disinfect the dermis and bring a fresh supply of blood to the surface of skin, helping the circulatory system to carry away unwanted debris. Base oils of camellia and jojoba bring super-emollience to the skin. Camellia is readily absorbed by the body, feeding and nourishing the skin, making it feel smoother and softer. Jojoba oil adds to the feeling of softness and brings a healthy and non-greasy shine to the skin. See page 21 for the **lemongrass blend** recipe.

Excess fat on upper arms

Too much fat on the upper arms probably occurs in tandem with too much fat on other parts of the body, and needs to be tackled as part of an overall body improvement regime. Either the **juniper blend** or the **lemongrass blend** can be used for massage. Allow your fingertips to detect the condition of the underlying skin – feel the lumps under the surface and encourage them to go away. If there are tiny spots or hard crystal-like deposits under the skin, encourage their removal and elimination by massage.

Flabby upper arms

We say that something is 'flabby' when it has lost its tone and has succumbed to the forces of gravity. Flabby upper arms are usually to be seen on women who have lost not only weight but also muscle tone, either from age or from crash dieting, allowing the skin to hang in folds. Some improvement in the appearance of the upper arms can be achieved with massage of the skin with **lemongrass blend**, followed by massage with **vetivert blend**. However, it will only be possible to effect a very gradual change in the condition and appearance of the skin, and best results will be achieved if a little light exercise is also incorporated.

Dry skin

Dry, wrinkly skin is the easist of the upper arm problems to rectify, as a dry skin denotes a lack of oils in the skin. Skin cells are constantly renewing themselves; as the old, dead cells are removed from the surface of our bodies, new cells are already being pushed upwards, towards the surface. By feeding the skin with pure oils , both essential and fatty, we can feed the deeper layers where the cells are formed, giving them the ideal conditions for birth and growth. Camellia oil and jojoba wax will give the skin all the nourishment it requires, whilst the **vetivert blend** will encourage the cells to absorb and retain moisture, making them plumper and more youthful.

Massage of upper arms

Whether your upper arm problem is cellulite, excess fat, flabby loose skin, or rough dry skin, the massage technique is the same. Massage of the upper arms, following an aromatic bath and skin brushing, is the most effective way to get essential oils into skin.

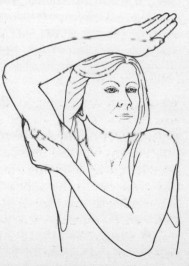

With your choice of massage blend, apply the oil to the upper left arm, from the elbow to the shoulder, covering all of the skin, underarm included. Rest the left wrist and hand across the top of the head – this will enable you to massage the underarm more easily. Using only your fingertips, smooth

Figure 19. Massaging the upper arms

and stroke the skin from the elbow to the armpit, with short and repetitive strokes, like sweeping leaves along the ground (see Figure 19). Be sensitive to your body and feel for any little fatty bumps, crystal or pimples under the surface, and massage these areas thoroughly. Apply more oil blend whenever necessary. Dropping your arm down by your side, massage the outer edge of your arm from elbow to shoulder, smoothing away the lumps and bumps. Make a mental note of any muscle soreness that you come across. Ask yourself whether the tenderness is due to physical strain of the triceps, such as driving, carrying a heavy bag, or exercising, or is it due to old toxins trapped in the tissues. If the latter, you will need to massage the area regularly until the toxins have been released and eliminated. Now turn the arm so that the palm is facing upwards, and massage the biceps. Again using fingertip massage, work the oil blend into the skin from elbow to shoulder. Finish by massaging the entire armpit area, and help your axillary glands to carry out their important function.

N.B. Do not shave, wax or use depilatory cream on the underarms immediately before or after massage of upper arms and under-arm area.

Elbows

It is often said that a woman's true age can be determined by looking at her elbows, because the elbows cannot be cosmetically enhanced and cared for in the way that the face can. But is this really true? Do we have to accept the inevitable gallop of age across our elbows when we take such great care to keep the signs of aging from our face?

We prop ourselves on an elbow to read a book, watch television, talk to a friend or lover, or merely to rest our head on one hand and watch the world go by. The elbow continues to support the weight of the upper body. And when working at a desk for long periods of time, the elbows are again used as a means of support to the upper body.

The flesh covering the elbow is, by necessity, fairly loose fitting, as elbows have to bend. It can therefore easily lose elasticity and become wrinkled. Whatever problem we experience with the condition of our elbows and upper arms, there is no magic solution that can be rubbed in before bedtime and cause a transformation by morning. Patience and effort are the only ways to make an improvement, both in the appearance and feel of the elbow.

Puffy fat elbows

Fat elbows are unlikely to be found in isolation, and will be part of an overall excess of adipose tissue in the body. The true solution lies in eating healthily and increasing the body's metabolism, but a useful aromatic adjunct is to massage the elbows with the **lemongrass blend** of oils. Lemongrass burns toxins in the connective tissue. The citrus oils of grapefruit and orange are cleansing and stimulating to the tissues, helping the lymph to take away fluids and proteins and return them to the circulatory system where they may be further broken down and eliminated from the body.

Massage of elbows

The main problems with the elbows are puffy or fat elbows and hard, dry and wrinkled skin. Although seemingly different, the cause is fairly constant – a build-up of toxins, fluids or fats due to inadequate lymph drainage and lack of physical care. Massage of the elbows and stimulation of the cubital lymph nodes (in the fold of the elbow) will help to bring about a more healthful, youthful appearance. Whatever our individual problem, the massage technique is the same.

Fingertip massage, using the chosen aromatic blend –

and lots of it – is required in the area of the elbow. Take a look at your elbows in a mirror. See what improvments need to take place and if you wish, make a note of the appearance of the elbows, so that you have a yardstick with which to measure progress. Massage of the elbows can be carried out whilst watching a favourite television programme but do protect clothing and furniture with towels before starting.

Pour a little blended oil into a small massage bowl or similar receptacle, for ease of use. Sit on the edge of your bed or chair with the left arm crossing in front of your body, and the left hand resting on the right thigh. Take up some massage oil with the fingers of your right hand and smooth into the skin around the elbow. If you are large chested, you may find it easier to lean forwards so that your left forearm is lying across your knees, and the breasts fall comfortably forward. Using fingertips, massage the flesh around the bony part of the elbow, feeling how much or how little flesh is covering the bone. Whilst smoothing in the oil, feel for any little bumps or hard spots under the surface of the skin. These are not supposed to be there and denote the presence of pockets of toxins, excess proteins, knotted fibres and crystal deposits. Now, with your fingertips, stroke and rub the skin on and around the elbow, giving extra attention to rough or lumpy areas. Continue the fingertip massage for about 15 minutes, or until your right hand feels tired. Then, stretching out your left arm so that the back of your hand is resting on your knees, massage the inner elbow where the cubital lymph nodes are housed. These nodes are responsible for the health of our forearms, hands and nails, filtering away poisons and producing lymphocytes. Using the flat of your hand stroke the flesh upwards from below the elbow to the top of the arm and finally spend a minute or so massaging the nodes at the top of the arm by lifting up the left arm and rubbing the nodes at the junction of the arm and the torso. Now change hands and massage the right arm in the same way.

Hard, dry and wrinkled elbows

As with dry upper arms, the problem of dry elbows is a lack of natural oil, which in mature skins is exacerbated by a breakdown in connective tissue and an inability to retain moisture. The blend of **vetivert in camellia** is a wonderful combination of essential and fatty oils for massaging dry, wrinkled elbows, since vetivert can help the skin cells to attract and hold water more easily. Sandalwood is another very useful oil for massaging into dry skin. Or try cleansing the elbows with a cotton wool pad soaked in **sandalwood aromatic water** and then massage in a little of the **vetivert in camellia**.

Neck

Whether long and sleek or short and thick, our neck supports our head, enables us to see around corners, and is a place of adornment. Like the elbows, the flesh covering the neck has to be fairly loose in order that we may have 180 degree flexibility to the left and right. The skin of the neck is a dense network of collagen fibres, intermingled with elastic fibres which enable the skin to stretch and then return to normal. Small enough to be encircled by our two hands, the neck houses an incredible collection of bones, veins, arteries, nerves, glands, lymph nodes and ducts, as well as the gullet and windpipe. The muscles of the neck have to support the weight of the head (around 4 kg) which is why too much strain or tension in the neck produces a headache.

Stretching the neck from time to time is beneficial to the muscles and the blood flow, and is especially important if our job causes us to sit for many hours a day with our heads facing in one direction, such as in front of a computer screen. Massaging the neck is also important for several reasons: to release tension from the muscles; to encourage the free flow of lymph, and the efficient drainage of waste products from the head, face and the neck itself; to allow good blood circulation; and to prevent any impingement of nerves. Looking after the neck is much more than just a cosmetic routine to enhance our physical beauty – it is a sensible way to keep the face, the head and the whole of the body in a good state of health.

Lines and loose skin

The neck should ideally be cleansed and moisturized every night as part of the daily care plan for the face (see Chapter 4). The skin on the neck, like the skin of the face, is subject to contact with polluted air and the elements, and will need to be thoroughly cleansed every day. After cleansing, apply the **vetivert in camillia** blend and using large, firm sweeps, massage into the sides of the neck using clean hands. With long hair pinned up, massage the back of the neck, from the hairline down to the shoulders, and rub away at any sore spots your fingers may discover. There are many lymph nodes in the neck which draw off toxins from the face and head.

Astringent mask

Just as an egg white mask with rose oil is astringent and toning for the face, it is equally beneficial for the neck. Whisk the white of a small or medium egg until frothy, then add one drop of rose absolute. Whisk again until the rose is incorporated and then spread the mask over your entire neck. Allow the mask to dry and wash it off when the skin begins to feel tight. Use cotton wool pads to remove all traces of mask. Pat the skin dry and whilst still damp, apply a little Vitamin E oil.

Neck massage

Ideally the front of the neck should be cleansed and massaged everyday at the same time as your face. In this way the skin stands the very best chance of retaining its elasticity, and staying free from lines. However, the back of the neck will only need to be massaged periodically, such as when you have a headache, or prior to an important function when you will be wearing your hair up and want your neck and shoulders to look as good as your face.

By massaging the back of the neck with a massage oil blend, we can release a lot of tension, relax sore and tight muscles, and encourage the dispersion of toxins and static energy, so easily accumulated by hours of desk work, driving, worrying over problems, or even just by sleeping in the wrong position at night.

Choose your favourite essential oil, or one of the following: lavender, myrtle, clary sage, geranium, rose, sandalwood, bergamot or patchouli.

Using one or two drops of essential oil in one teaspoon fatty oil, apply a little mixture to the fingertips and place your hands on the back of your neck so that your fingers meet on the vertebral column (see Figure 20). Now draw the fingers down, round and up so that the neck is being covered in large circles, and continue to do this for as long as you feel comfortable. Next, stretch hands even further down the back of the neck, and starting

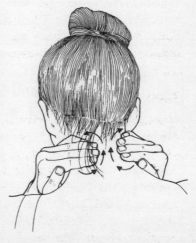

Figure 20. Massaging the neck

at the spine and applying firm pressure, draw your fingers round the bottom of your neck until they reach the right angle between neck and shoulder.

Repeat this move several times as it is a very effective way of removing tension and allows energy to flow to the head. Next, place fingertips at base of neck and slide them up the back of the neck, with fingers on either side of the spine. When your fingers reach the hairline, apply stronger pressure and hold for a count of five. Allow your fingers to press and soothe all sore spots along the occiput (where the skull joins the neck) and continue outwards until your hands reach your ears. Then, taking the back of the neck between fingers and thumb, squeeze gently, allowing your fingers and thumb to slide across the skin and meet at the spinal column. Finish the massage by stroking the fingers from the top to the bottom of the neck, ending by sweeping hands round to front of the neck and applying firm pressure to the lymph nodes below the clavicle.

Back and Shoulder Plan

Day	1	2	3	4	5	6	7	8	9	10	11	12	13	14
Bathe and skin brush	✓	✓	✓	✓	✓	✓	✓	✓	✓	✓	✓	✓	✓	✓
Massage upper arms	✓		✓		✓		✓		✓		✓		✓	
Massage elbows	✓		✓		✓		✓		✓		✓		✓	
Massage neck		✓					✓					✓		
Neck mask				✓						✓				

Chapter 12

Knees, ankles and feet

The problems: Fat knees; puffy knees; wrinkly knees. Puffy ankles; hidden ankles; tired feet.

The causes: Poor metabolism; excess fat; dehydrated skin; age; neglect.

The solutions: Aromatic bathing; skin brushing; massage; foot bath.

Knees

Even a woman with the most shapely legs and gorgeous figure can feel let down by her knees, especially when her legs are bare. Fortunately the essential oils can work on a deep level in the skin of the knees, just as they can on the face or any other part of the body. The most common problems are fat knees, puffy-looking knees, or wrinkly knees and I lay claim to the latter. In all knee problems, aromatic bathing and skin brushing are the first step, followed by massage with a well chosen blend of essential and fatty oils.

Aromatic bathing and skin brushing

The choice of the oils here is not so crucial, so choose one you particularly enjoy. The emphasis is on skin brushing. Take your nail brush and brush up the leg from ankles to knees, using medium pressure. Then brush across and around the knee as well as underneath the knee where the

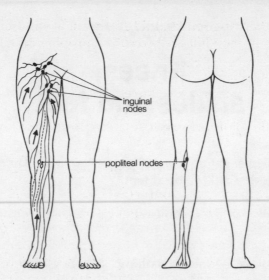

Figure 21. Lymph nodes of the knees and legs

popliteal lymph nodes lie. Next, bend the knee, and with firmer pressure, brush the top of the knee from all sides, and take the brush strokes about a third of the way up the thigh. Finish the skin brushing by stroking the bristles along the 'knicker line'.

The skin may look pink and feel hot, which is a good sign because blood is being brought to the surface of the skin. This has two effects: it brings nutrients to the skin surface and it prepares the skin for the essential oil massage.

Fat knees

A massage with the **lemongrass blend** is excellent for those with fat knees, as it decongests and detoxifies the area. Jojoba may also be used alone since it penetrates quickly and deeply into the skin and is able to emulsify fats very effectively.

Puffy knees

I recommend a massage with the **juniper blend** for any

woman who experiences fluid retention around the knees. This is a common but easily resolved problem so take heart.

Wrinkly knees

Age and dry skin produce knees that look a little wrinkled. Like wrinkles on the face, a firm massage with the **vetivert in camellia** blend can restore a youthful, firm texture to these trouble spots.

Massage of the knees

For any problem, sit comfortably and with your chosen blend, massage the entire knee area. Then, using finger-tips, feel for any little knots, lumps, toxic deposits or unwanted fat. Massage your knee in small circular movements from below the kneecap to about a third of the way up the thigh (see Figure 22). With both thumbs placed on the leg above the knee, work outwards and downwards towards the back of the knees and the lymph nodes. Continue for up to 15 minutes per knee or if your fingers tire, for as long as possible.

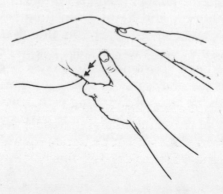

Figure 22. Massage of the knees

Ankles and feet

Being even further from the torso than the knees, the ankles and feet can easily accumulate fluids (especially when pre-menstrual), fats and toxins.

Foot baths and skin brushing

Virtually any of the essential oils mentioned in this book can be used in a foot bath. In the summertime, peppermint is very cooling as it contains natural menthol. In the winter my choice of oil is myrtle, as it is comforting and warming. Any woman who suffers from foot odour could use cypress, juniper or frankincense, since these oils all have natural deodorant properties.

With a nail brush, brush the top of the foot from the toes to the ankle, paying particular attention to the area around the inside and outside of the ankle bone. Most of the lymph from the foot drains to the popliteal nodes, but some lymph vessels go directly to the inguinal nodes. Therefore, stimulate both areas with the nail brush.

Pufffy ankles

A massage with the **juniper blend** is wonderfully effective as juniper is a diuretic and helps drain fluid from this area. Some women, and I am no exception, find that after a party or other occasion when larger than normal quantities of alcohol have been consumed, the ankles become a little puffy – this is the body's way of saying it is having difficulty in coping with the alcohol. Drinking extra glasses of water is a valuable aid to your body's eliminative system, as is a massage with a diuretic essential oil.

Hidden ankles

You can either massage with the **lemongrass blend** or jojoba oil to help uncover ankle bones you had forgotten you had.

Massage of the ankles and feet

Sit comfortably on a chair with your legs crossed and apply the chosen oils to the top and sides of one foot and ankle, or sit on top of your bed with one foot resting on a towel and your knee bent upwards. With firm fingertip pressure, stroke from the toes to the ankle, and then draw your fingers around the ankle. Continue these movements for several minutes. Apply the maximum pressure you find bearable; some of us have very sensitive feet and ankles, but the massage should have a degree of firmness. If the feet and ankles are massaged on a regular basis, they do become less tender to the touch as toxins and fluids are removed. Finish the massage by smoothing the skin up to the knees, so that the lymph is encouraged to drain. As some lymph vessels drain directly into the inguinal nodes, be sure to massage this area as well. Many women experience swelling and tenderness of the flesh just below the ankle bone immediately prior to menstruation, and gentle massage of this area will help the body to release tissue fluids.

Tired feet

Lots of tension is stored in the feet, not to mention the trauma of teetering around on high heels, or simply standing on and using our relatively tiny feet. They need a treat from time to time. Nothing is lovelier than an aromatic foot soak. Place your feet in a few inches of warm water in the bottom of your bath tub or in a separate bowl to which a few drops of essential oil have been added – lavender, geranium, ylang-ylang, rose, bergamot, the choice is yours.

After a 10 minutes soak, use a pumice stone to smooth away dry skin from the heels and toes. Cover one knee with a towel and put your other foot up for a massage. Clench your fist and, starting at the base of the toes, draw your knuckles along the length of the foot to the heel (see

Figure 23). Cover the whole foot with knuckle caresses which stimulate many foot reflex points and release tension. Change towel to opposite knee and tend your other foot. Dry feet with a towel and apply a little **rose in camellia** or a little jojoba oil. You should feel as though you are walking on air!

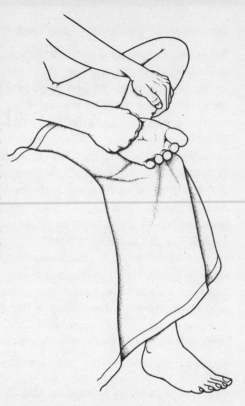

Figure 23. Massage for tired feet

Knees, Ankles and Feet Plan													
Day	1	2	3	4	5	6	7	8	9	10	11	12	13	14
Bathe and skin brush	✓	✓	✓	✓	✓	✓	✓	✓	✓	✓	✓	✓	✓	✓
Knee massage	✓		✓		✓		✓		✓		✓		✓	
Foot bath				✓				✓				✓		
Ankle and foot massage				✓				✓				✓		

Chapter 13

Hand and nail care

The problems: Dry skin; dehydrated skin; fat or puffy hands; brittle nails; ridged nails.

The causes: Lack of moisture; insufficient sebum production; environment; diet.

The solutions: Aromatic hand baths; nail soaks; moisturizing; massage; barrier cream.

Hands

Hands and face are the two areas of our body most often exposed to the elements and whilst we protect our facial skin with moisturizers and make-up, our hands are often neglected and become damaged. As there is only a thin layer of flesh over the bones of the hand, the backs of our hands can age more quickly than the skin of the face, so that even if we are blessed with a youthful-looking face, our hands can instantly reveal our true age.

There are two ways to improve your hands.

1. A barrier cream that can be applied regularly throughout the day.
2. Nightly moisturizing routine with rejuvenating oils and aromatic waters, followed by the donning of white cotton gloves for the night (optional).

Daytime barrier cream

A barrier cream has two functions. One is to provide an invisible film or barrier against the environment – the weather, central heating, water in all its usages (washing up, washing our hair, handling the laundry), etc. The second is to soften and moisturize dry skin and to feed it with nourishing fatty oils and essential oils.

Beeswax, jojoba oil, camellia oil, water and essential oils are the ingredients necessary to make an emollient and protective hand cream which is very inexpensive. Being simple to make, and not containing any preservatives, it is preferable to make a batch every three to four weeks, rather than make a large quantity and hope that it will still be as fresh in six months' time. Even when using the non-oxidizing oils of jojoba and camellia, there will be a gradual breakdown in the consistency and freshness of the cream because of the addition of water, and it will not keep for a long period of time. Commercially available hand creams must, by law, contain enough preservatives to guarantee a shelf-life of 18 months. Although preservatives are not beneficial to the condition of the skin, they serve a useful purpose which is to inhibit the growth of bacteria. As we are making batches of cream without the use of preservatives, it is important to remember this, and always to include the 'date of manufacture' on the pot's label.

There is a huge range of essential oils which could be chosen for their fragrance as well as for their ability to soften and protect the skin, for example, lemon and orange or bergamot and orange. Warm, earthy aromas make a pleasing bouquet when blended, such as vetivert and rose or patchouli and ylang-ylang or sandalwood and rose. The final choice will rest with you – if you are not happy with the aroma it is unlikely that you will want to apply the cream throughout the day.

The barrier cream recipe can be found on page 26. This cream is pure, fresh, fragranced to your preference, incredibly cheap to make, almost as simple as making an omelette – and much more fun.

Night time rejuvenating hand massage

Having experimented with various combinations of fatty oils and waxes, essential oil blends and aromatic waters, the combination that I find most effective is **vetivert in camellia** and **sandalwood aromatic water**.

Massage the hands before going to bed using **vetivert in camellia**. Hold your left hand with your right, and with the right thumb massage the back of the hand, using small circular movements and working between the carpel bones (see Figure 24). Take one finger of your left hand between

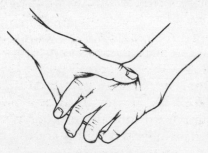

Figure 24. Massaging the hands

the fingers and thumb of your right hand and massage the entire length of the finger. Rub your palms together and smooth the oil into the entire hand and wrist. Repeat on other hand. Next, pour a little **sandalwood aromatic water** into the palm of one hand. Carefully rub the aromatic water into both hands, as if you were washing your hands. When dry, apply a little more **vetivert in camellia** and a little more **sandalwood aromatic water**. Keep applying a little more

sandalwood aromatic water and **vetivert in camellia** until your hands cannot absorb any more. After massaging the hands, spend a few minutes massaging the lymph nodes situated in the elbow area (see Figure 25).

A pair of cotton gloves, if worn all night, will enhance the penetrating action of the oils. This treatment is guaranteed to soften and improve the condition of even the most neglected pair of hands.

Hand bath

Hands that are dry, rough or damaged can be healed and softened by the use of an aromatic hand bath. Any of the essential oils which are beneficial for dry skin may be used, such as lavender, geranium, sandalwood, rose, vetivert, frankincense or patchouli.

You will need a bowl that is large enough to place your hands in for half an hour; a casserole dish may prove to be the correct size. Seat yourself comfortably and place first a hand towel and then the bowl of aromatic liquid on your lap.

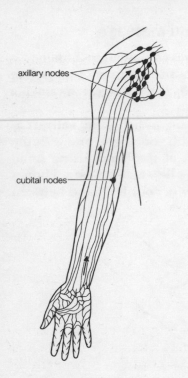

axillary nodes

cubital nodes

Figure 25. Lymph vessels and nodes of the hands and arms

Essential oils differ in their ability to disperse in water and if using one of the viscous oils – rose, sandalwood vetivert or patchouli – it will first be necessary to mix them with a thinner oil such as lavender, orange or myrtle.

Place essential oils in the bowl, add warm water and allow your hands to soak for 10-15 minutes.

1 drop vetivert   or 2 drops rose
1 drop sandalwood   2 drops lavender
2 drops lemon or bergamot   2 drops bergamot

Pat hands dry with a clean towel and apply a liberal amount of jojoba oil. Massage into the hands, as if washing your hands with the oil, until your hands have absorbed as much jojoba as possible. Rub excess oil onto any other area of dry skin such as the elbows or knees, or alternatively blot the excess with a tissue.

The nails

The nail is composed of keratin, as is the skin, and is a horny plate of the epidermis. It consists of cornified scales, overlapping like roof tiles. The nail bed is the living part

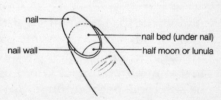

Figure 26. The nail

of the nail and consists of connective tissue channels that carry blood vessels along the nail's length, from the half moon to the fingertip. It is the flow of blood beneath the surface of the nail which gives the pink or red tinge. The nail projecting from the finger tip is completely dead, which enables us to cut and file our nails without experiencing pain (see Figure 26).

Most women like to have attractively shaped nails which are strong, smooth and enhance the sense of touch. Whatever our preferred length, if we break a nail, we immediately experience a loss of sensitivity. Our sense of touch has been diminished.

Nothing much can be done to increase the strength of the nail once it has grown beyond the fingertip, but much can be done to grow healthy nails in the nail bed. When nails are dry and brittle and split easily, it is simply because they are not receiving sufficient 'food' in order for them to grow. The aromatic way to bring nutrients to the nail bed is to use a hypereamic oil, such as myrtle, either in the form of a massage oil or as a nail soak.

Massage oil for nails

A simple but effective massage oil for nails can be prepared in minutes.

1 teaspoon jojoba oil
5-6 drops myrtle oil

Add myrtle to jojoba and stir until mixed. Dip the fingertips into the mixture so that some oil goes under the nail. Next, massage the oil into the nail wall, half moon and up to the first joint of the finger. When myrtle mixture has begun to be absorbed, put your fingertips together so that your hands form a sphere, and gently press the nails of the right hand underneath the nails of the left hand. Hold for a few seconds. Then press the nails of the left hand under the nails of the right hand.

Such intensive nail care is probably unnecessary if you are massaging face, head or body on a daily basis, since the nails automatically become more healthy and grow faster when hands come into contact with essential oils.

Aromatic nail soak

An alternative to using the massage oil for the nails is to soak the fingertips in a pot of warm water.

2 drops lavender oil
2 drops niaouli oil
3 drops Vitamin E oil (optional)

Place the oils in a small bowl (a breakfast bowl is ideal) and
add a few drops of liquid soap so that an emulsion will be
formed when the water is added. Half-fill the bowl with
comfortably warm water and immerse the fingertips of both
hands in the aromatic liquid.

Both lavender and niaouli are tissue stimulants, and
promote the growth of new skin – one of the reasons why
they are used to heal burns. By soaking the fingertips in this
aromatic liquid (especially if Vitamin E is included), a highly
nutritious meal is provided for our nails. Allow nails to soak
for 10-20 minutes, depending on how starved your nails are.
Rinse your hands in clear water after soaking, pat dry, and
massage in a little jojoba oil or aromatic barrier cream.

Hand and Nail Care Plan

Day	1	2	3	4	5	6	7	8	9	10	11	12	13	14
Night time hand massage	✓	✓	✓	✓	✓	✓	✓	✓	✓	✓	✓	✓	✓	✓
Daily use of barrier cream	✓	✓	✓	✓	✓	✓	✓	✓	✓	✓	✓	✓	✓	✓
Hand bath			✓						✓					✓
Nail massage			✓						✓					✓
Nail soak	✓						✓						✓	

Chapter 14

Don't forget...

As there is no real beauty without health and vitality, it's important to follow those commonsense guidelines to good living that we so commonly forget. Without them, we find ourselves taking three steps forward and two steps back. To maximize the returns from your investment in the 14-day aromabeauty plan, be sure to take good care of all of you, not just for two weeks but for every day of the year.

Rest

Don't forget the importance of sleep. It is generally accepted that adults require eight hours of sleep to function at their best. It is only during the hours of sleep that the immune system repairs itself. Like a trusted watchman, the immune system is on guard and working on our behalf during waking hours, but at night while we rest, it can replenish and ready itself for the next day's demands. The immune system is our protector and friend and we must understand and respect its needs.

Nerve force or vital energy is something we can only regenerate by adequate rest and refreshing sleep. We can burn up our resources of energy and dip into the reserves, but when this is used up we are completely spent. If we can repay the borrowed energy with periods of rest and respite there is no problem, but if we continue to use the daily amount of allocated energy as well as taking from the reserves, then we become bankrupt.

A restful night's sleep is essential for good health (see

page 60). I make it a habit not to take my troubles to bed with me. Easier said than done? For me, writing down my problems before bed allows me to let go of them for the night. This, followed by an aromatic bath with lavender, geranium or rose oil, always does the trick. After a particularly stressful day, I may also put a few drops of lavender or rose oil on my electric fragrancer.

Diet

Don't forget to eat sensibly. Years ago, before freezers and convenience foods became commonplace, we ate vegetables and fruits, grains and cereals, and natural proteins. It's strange that we now classify this as a wholefood diet whereas in those days it was the norm. Let's get back to basics. Our bodies need good fuel to function properly. Too many refined and denatured foods are also a major cause of excess free oxygen radicals in the body. These oxygen radicals generally bind to carbon or hydrogen atoms and are excreted from our bodies as carbon dioxide or water, but when they cannot find a source to bind with, oxygen radicals can create chaos throughout the body and lead to cellular breakdown. This is now known to be a primary cause of cellulite, in which fat cells damaged by free radicals become vulnerable to invasion from toxins and water. Many illnesses can be attributed to excess free radicals in the body.

Don't forget to incorporate unsaturated fatty acids into your diet. While saturated fats (mainly from animals) are the bad guys that raise cholesterol levels and cause obesity, unsaturated fats are the good guys that are essential for healthy skin. Even a mild deficiency can cause skin dryness and premature ageing. The main source of unsaturated fatty acids is vegetable oils, such as soyabean, sesame and sunflower oils, but the best source is virgin olive oil.

Water

Don't forget to drink plenty of water. Due to an often unsatis-
factory diet, centrally heated housing and stressful lifestyle,
the body easily becomes dehydrated and it is very important to drink extra water. This not only helps keep the skin
supple but flushes out harmful toxins. I recommend that
during the 14-day beauty plan you drink at least six glasses
of water a day in order to dilute and transport the toxins
released from the tissues. Like a teapot full of tea leaves
being tipped into a kitchen sink and being washed down
the plughole, we need to dilute the poisons with water
before they can be efficiently dealt with by the lymphatic
system. It is via the lymph nodes that unwanted substances
are broken down and filtered into the blood stream and
then excreted from the body via the normal channels. Each
bean-shaped lymph node is connected to other lymph
nodes by a network of lymphatic vessels. Afferent lymphatic
vessels empty their contents into the node whilst efferent
vessels carry lymph away from the node. Because there are
several vessels leading into the node and only one vessel
leading out, there is always the possibility of a 'bottleneck'
situation, or a traffic jam. Traffic jams are never permanent
but whilst they last they can be inconvenient and uncom-
fortable. In a similar way, we may experience this discomfort
as tenderness at the site of the nodes when the body is
trying to rid itself of toxins as can happen when we fast,
exercise rigorously or massage an area of cellulite.

I only drink bottled or purified water, as I consider tap
water not only unpalatable but hazardous to my health.
What should be the purest form of refreshment has become
a cocktail of bacteria, industrial wastes and chemicals such
as aluminium, lead, nitrates and chlorine. Chlorine, which
gives our tapwater its distinctive smell, can create free radicals when taken into the body, as well as tasting foul.

Vitamins

Don't forget to supplement your diet with vitamins and minerals. If we always ate well-balanced and healthy foods, there would be no necessity for multi-vitamins and mineral supplements except in times of illness or stress. However, because most of us live very hectic lives, I do recommend a multi-vitamin/mineral supplement taken at breakfast time. I recommend extra Vitamin C during the winter months when our consumption of fresh fruit and raw vegetables is down. Vitamin C is vital for strong healthy cells and counteracts the effects of free radicals in the body.

During times of stress, taking B-Complex is an excellent way to replenish the supply of B vitamins burnt up by mental activity. I have found that in times of crisis, when the adrenal glands are working overtime, a course of Vitamin B5 (pantothenic acid) helps me feel calmer as B5 regulates the function of the adrenal glands (which govern the output of more than 40 hormones, including adrenaline).

Exercise

Don't forget to exercise. Regular exercise, like a sensible diet, keeps the body in good working order. Drastic exercise programmes that attempt to burn off excess years of sedentary living overnight are as dangerous (and impossible) as crash diets. Exercise not only strengthens and tones the muscles, but also regulates the flow of lymph, improves the functioning of the cardiovascular system and burns off calories. I live in the middle of nowhere, so my exercise is running up and down stairs. It doesn't matter what you do, as long as you do it routinely.

Don't forget the old adage, everything in moderation. Maybe this sounds boring, as we all remember the memorable moments of excess. But in general be kind to your body. I have a particular fondness for champagne and I love a glass of white wine with dinner, but I'm aware that alcohol in excess is poisonous. It can damage the liver, dehydrate the skin, and speed up the visible signs of ageing. The current recommendation is that women limit their alcohol consumption to nine drinks a week. One drink equals half a pint of beer or one measure of spirit or one glass of table wine or one small glass of sherry.

Tea and coffee are also relatively toxic in large quantities. Having a warm drink with a friend or neighbour is a pleasant social ritual, which I wouldn't want to give up, but it's not good sense to take in large quantities of tannin and caffeine.

Don't forget: no smoking. While most of the pleasures of life can be yours if used in moderation, smoking is one definite exception. I strongly advocate against smoking cigarettes. Not only can it kill you, it can accelerate the ageing process by damaging the DNA content of cells. Smoking is a true poison that at the very least robs us of our beauty by creating premature wrinkles and dry sallow skin.

Don't forget to protect your skin from the harmful ultraviolet rays of the sun. Nothing is lovelier than sitting in the fresh air on a sunny day. It lightens the spirit and enriches us with Vitamin D. But here, too, over-indulgence is detrimental as sunbathing burns and destroys the cells of the skin. Far from the stereotype of the bronzed beauty, prolonged and regular exposure to the harsh rays of the sun dries out, blemishes and ages the skin. I'd quite like to bring back parasols as a fashion accessory, but until that day I'll sit in the shade.

And finally, *don't forget* to smile. The world is filled with hardships, and we all have our problems and stresses, but in the busy confusion of life, do take time to smell the roses.

Chapter 15

The 14-day
body blitz

Getting married. Going on holiday. Just met that special man, and want to look and feel your best. Your child has started school and you have time to yourself. Whatever the reason, if you want to improve the shape, tone and health of your body, follow the 14-Day Aromabeauty Body Blitz chart.

The chart contains suggestions for improving the whole body by dedicating one or two hours a day of your time. If you have less time or don't have a problem with a particular body area, then delete a section which is not of interest.

Days 1-14 are planned so that by the end of the two-week period, every problem area has been worked on. However, these are only my suggestions and you can easily swop around the individual tasks from one day to another. Some tasks, such as massage of the thighs and buttocks crop up everyday, as these body areas are subject to the most self-criticism, and almost every woman would like to improve her thighs and buttocks. Massage of the breasts also crops up everyday, as I believe that preventative measures need to be taken to ensure healthy breasts stay that way. All other regimes are interspersed throughout the 14 days.

General body blitz

The following day plans are in addition to the everyday beauty activities (see Chapter 4) which include aromatic bathing, skin brushing, cleansing and moisturizing of the face, and hand care.

Day 1

Thigh massage – lemongrass blend	30 mins
Friction of back (in bath)	5 mins
Self-massage (neck and shoulders)	10 mins
Rejuvenating face routine	15 mins
Solar plexus massage	5 mins
Breast massage	5 mins
Hair treatment (massage)	10 mins +
(+ 1-2 hours hair wrapped in towel)	
Time needed	**1 hr 20 mins**

Day 2

Thigh massage – jojoba or camellia	15 mins
Buttock massage – lemongrass blend	30 mins
Face mask	10 mins
Nail soak and massage	15 mins
Breast massage	5 mins
Time needed	**1 hr 15 mins**

Day 3

Head massage	15 mins
Thigh massage – jojoba or camellia	20 mins
Buttock massage – lemongrass blend	20 mins
Eye compress	15 mins
Tummy massage	15 mins
Breast massage	5 mins
Time needed	**1 hr 30 mins**

Day 4

Thigh massage – lemongrass blend	20 mins
Buttock massage – jojoba or camellia	20 mins
Rejuvenating face routine	15 mins
Friction of back (in bath)	5 mins

Knee massage	10 mins
Breast massage	5 mins
Time needed	**1 hr 15 mins**

Day 5

Thigh massage – jojoba or camellia	15 mins
Buttock massage – jojoba or camellia	15 mins
Massage of upper arms and elbows	20 mins
Breast massage	5 mins
Tummy massage	10 mins
(+ time for cling-film wrap)	
Time needed	**1 hr 5 mins**

Day 6

Thigh massage – jojoba or camellia	20 mins
Buttock massage – juniper blend	20 mins
Neck massage	10 mins
Breast massage	5 mins
Foot bath	15 mins
Hand bath (can be done at	
same time as footbath)	15 mins
Ankle and foot massage	15 mins
Time needed	**1 hr 25 mins**

Day 7

Thigh massage – juniper blend	20 mins
Buttock massage – jojoba or camellia	15 mins
Face mask	15 mins
Breast masssage	5 mins
Friction of back (in bath)	5 mins
Tummy massage	20 mins
Time needed	**1 hr 20 mins**

Day 8

Thigh massage – jojoba or camellia	15 mins
Buttock massage – lemongrass blend	15 mins
Rejuvenating face routine	15 mins
Breast massage	5 mins
Self-massage – shoulders	10 mins
Solar plexus massage	5 mins
Hair treatment	10 mins +
(+ time needed for hair wrap)	
Time needed	**1 hr 15 mins**

Day 9

Thigh massage – jojoba or camellia	15 mins
Buttock massage – lemongrass blend	15 mins
Massage upper arms and elbows	20 mins
Breast massage	5 mins
Knee massage	10 mins
Nail soak and massage	15 mins
Time needed	**1 hr 20 mins**

Day 10

Head massage	10 mins
Thigh massage – juniper blend	15 mins
Buttock massage – jojoba or camellia	10 mins
Eye compress	15 mins
Neck massage	10 mins
Breast massage	5 mins
Friction of back (in bath)	5 mins
Time needed	**1 hr 10 mins**

Day 11

Thigh massage – jojoba or camellia	20 mins
Buttock massage – jojoba or camellia	20 mins
Rejuvenating face routine	15 mins

Breast massage	5 mins
Knee massage	10 mins
Time needed	**1 hr 10 mins**

Day 12

Thigh massage – jojoba or camellia	15 mins
Buttock massage – juniper blend	15 mins
Massage of upper arms and elbows	20 mins
Breast massage	5 mins
Tummy massage	20 mins
(+ time for cling-film wrap)	
Time needed	**1 hr 15 mins**

Day 13

Thigh massage – vetivert in camellia	10 mins
Buttock massage – vetivert in camellia	10 mins
Face mask	10 mins
Breast massage	5 mins
Friction of back (in bath)	5 mins
Knee massage	10 mins
Back pack	30 mins
Time needed	**1 hr 20 mins**

Day 14

Thigh massage – vetivert in camellia	10 mins
Buttock massage – vetivert in camellia	10 mins
Rejuvenating face routine	15 mins
Neck massage	10 mins
Breast massage	5 mins
Self-massage – shoulders	10 mins
Solar plexus massage	5 mins
Hand bath	15 mins
Hair treatment	10 mins +
(+ time of 1-2 hours for hair wrap)	
Time needed	**1 hr 30 mins**

Esssential oils blends, when required, are listed alongside the daily activity. e.g. 'Day 1. Thigh massage – lemongrass blend' indicates that you should use the **lemongrass blend** which can be found in Chapter 3. Where there is no recommended blend, you can choose which of the ready-blended oils to use, or which essences and fatty base to blend yourself.

General Body Blitz Plan

Day	1	2	3	4	5	6	7	8	9	10	11	12	13	14
Face														
Rejuvenating massage routine	✓			✓				✓			✓			✓
Mask		✓				✓						✓		
Eye compress			✓							✓				
Hair and Head														
Oil treatment	✓							✓						✓
Head massage			✓							✓		✓		
Breasts														
Massage	✓	✓	✓	✓	✓	✓	✓	✓	✓	✓	✓	✓	✓	✓
Back and Shoulders														
Friction in bath	✓			✓			✓			✓			✓	
Back pack													✓	
Self massage	✓							✓						✓
Tummy and waist														
Massage			✓		✓	✓						✓		
Cling-film wrap					✓							✓		
Solar plexus massage	✓							✓						✓

Day	1	2	3	4	5	6	7	8	9	10	11	12	13	14
Thighs														
Massage with lemongrass	✓			✓										
Massage with juniper						✓			✓					
Massage with vetivert in camellia													✓	✓
Massage with jojoba or camellia		✓	✓		✓	✓		✓	✓		✓	✓		
Buttocks														
Massage with lemongrass		✓	✓					✓	✓					
Massage with juniper						✓					✓			
Massage with vetivert in camellia													✓	✓
Massage with jojoba or camellia				✓	✓		✓			✓	✓			
Upper arms, elbows and neck														
Massage arms/elbows					✓				✓			✓		
Massage neck						✓			✓					✓
Knees, ankles and feet														
Knee massage				✓					✓		✓		✓	
Foot bath						✓								
Ankle and foot massage						✓								
Hands and nails														
Hand bath						✓								✓
Nail/hand massage		✓							✓					
Nail soak		✓							✓					

Chapter 16

Compendium of oils

Part A: Essential oils

BERGAMOT *(Citrus Bergamia)*
Family: *Rutaceae*

Plant: Tree
Part used: Peel of fruit
Extraction: Cold expression
Fragrance: Spicy, citrus

A lovely pale green oil, bergamot is refreshing and uplifting. It is cleansing not only for the body but also for the mind and spirit. One of the most frequently used oils to reduce tension and stress, bergamot has a unique balancing effect. In beauty care its primary role is in combating oily skin, spots and acne.
Cautionary note: Bergamot is not to be used prior to sunbathing or using a sunbed as the skin may become more sensitive to burning and possible pigmentation.

Aromabeauty care
Bath p.m. • Facial care • Lip balm • Hair care • Hand care • Massage oil • Body compress • Vaporiser

CLARY SAGE *(Salvia Scarea)*
Family: *Labiateae*

Plant: Herb
Part used: Flowering tops and leaves
Extraction: Steam distillation
Fragrance: Clear herbal-floral

This clear, non-viscous oil has a powerfully uplifting effect, even to the point of euphoria. Clary sage eliminates tension and releases sensuality. In beauty care it is cleansing and antiseptic, as well as soothing to inflammed skin. An effective moisturizer, clary sage is particularly beneficial for dry or mature skin.

Aromabeauty care
Bath a.m. • Bath p.m. • Facial care • Hand care • Massage oil • Vaporiser

FRANKINCENSE *(Boswellia Carterii/Thurifera)*
Family: *Burseraceae*

Plant: Tree
Part used: Resin from trunk
Extraction: Steam distillation
Fragrance: Balsamic

A beautiful golden oil, frankincense has been used for millenia to enhance spiritual awareness and harmony. Very relaxing and soothing, the oil is also strengthening in times of need. In beauty care, it is a gentle but powerful astringent and tonic for the skin. Frankincense is the oil par excellence for mature skin as it helps renew and regenerate skin cells, smoothing away wrinkles.

Aromabeauty Care
Bath p.m. • Facial care • Hand care • Massage oil • Vaporiser

GERANIUM *(Pelargonium Graveolens/Roseum)*
Family: *Geraniaceae*

Plant: Flowering shrub
Part used: Flowers and leaves
Extraction: Steam distillation
Fragrance: Sweet and fresh

With its delightful lingering aroma, geranium is one of nature's most versatile essences. Termed a balancing oil, it is both uplifting and sedative depending on your needs, and is thus highly effective in reducing stress. In beauty care, geranium's balancing action make it suitable for dry or greasy skin. It is also a marvellous skin cleanser and toner.

Aromabeauty care
Bath a.m. • Bath p.m. • Facial care • Lip balm • Hair care • Hand care • Massage oil • Vaporiser

GRAPEFRUIT *(Citrus Paradisi)*
Family: *Rutaceae*

Plant: Tree
Part used: Peel of fruit
Extraction: Cold expression
Fragrance: Bitter, citrousy aroma

Grapefruit is a lovely citrus oil that provides a zesty and refreshing lift when energy is low. Uplifting to the emotions, grapefruit is a gentle tonic that counterbalances the effects of stress. In beauty care, its stimulant effects are evidenced by grapefruit's remarkable detoxifying properties, making it ideal in the treatment of cellulite and obesity. The oil is similarly beneficial at decongesting, toning and cleansing the skin, as well as in regulating the production of sebum, and is thus effective in reducing the oiliness of the hair and scalp.

Aromabeauty Care
Bath a.m. • Facial care • Hair care • Massage oil • Vaporiser

JUNIPER *(Juniperus Communis)*
Family: *Cupressaceae*

Plant: Bush
Part used: Berry
Extraction: Steam distillation
Fragrance: Fresh, outdoor aroma

The aroma of juniper is bracing and strengthening and the oil is excellent for overcoming mental and physical fatigue. Its effects on the emotions are similarly stimulating and uplifting. In beauty care, the antiseptic and astringent properties of juniper make it ideal for treating acne as well as oily and congested skin. Juniper is renowned as a detoxifying oil that helps in the elimination of cellulite.

Aromabeauty care
Bath a.m. • Facial care • Hair care • Massage oil • Vaporiser

LAVENDER *(Lavandula Angustifolia)*
Family: *Labiatae*

Plant: Flowering shrub
Plant used: Flowering stems and leaves
Extraction: Steam distillation
Fragrance: Clean, sharp floral fragrance

Perhaps the most popular essential oil in use today, lavender possesses remarkable healing powers, and its versatility is unparalleled. On an emotional sphere, it is primarily sedative and calming and thus frequently used to release stress and promote sleep. In beauty care, lavender's action on the skin makes it beneficial for all skin types. Well known for its antiseptic and soothing properties, lavender is an excellent choice for problem skin and sun burn. It is also a wonderful oil for mature skin as it stimulates cellular renewal thus helping to keep skin young-looking.

Aromabeauty care
Bath p.m. • Facial care • Hair care • Hand care • Massage oil • Body compress • Vaporiser

LEMON *(Citrus Limonum)*
Family: *Rutaceae*

Plant: Tree
Part used: Peel of fruit

Extraction: Cold expression
Fragrance: Zesty, refreshing

Lemon oil is stimulating and invigorating, and acts to sharpen the mind and restore or increase vitality. This pale yellow or green coloured oil is a refreshing tonic that helps lift the spirits and strengthen reserve. In beauty care, lemon oil is commonly employed to decongest and cleanse a greasy scalp or oily and problem skin. Lemon is also a natural detoxifying agent, making it valuable in the treatment of cellulite.

Cautionary note: Lemon is not to be used prior to sunbathing or using a sunbed as the skin may become more sensitive to burning and possible pigmentation. The oil should always be used fresh; discard if cloudy.

Aromabeauty care
Bath a.m. • Facial care • Lip balm • Hair care • Hand care • Massage oil • Vaporiser

LEMONGRASS *(Cymbopogan Citratus)*
Family: *Graminaceae*

Plant: Grass
Part used: Stem amd leaves
Extraction: Steam distillation
Fragrance: Strong and lemony

Mentally stimulating and emotionally strengthening, lemongrass is one of the best essential oils for revitalizing a tired constitution. Ayurvedic medicine of India has used lemongrass for thousands of years to dispel toxins, especially bacteria. In beauty care, this makes lemongrass oil invaluable in the treatment of obesity and cellulite, caused by an accumulation of toxins lodged in the tissues.

Cautionary note: Exercise restraint when using lemongrass oil as it is very powerful and may irritate the skin. In a bath, use no more than three drops well dispersed in the water.

Lemongrass oil in very weak concentration is generally best reserved for massage blends.

Aromabeauty Care
Bath a.m. • Massage oil • Vaporiser

MYRTLE *(Myrtus Communis)*
Family: *Myrtaceae*

Plant: Flowering shrub
Part used: Leaves
Extraction: Steam distillation
Fragrance: Warm and spicy

A warm, sensual and enveloping fragrance, myrtle has been used since Greco-Roman times as a symbol of love and a general aphrodisiac. While soothing and mildly sedative for the body, it also possesses the ability to lift the emotions and allow positive feelings to flow. In beauty care, myrtle is excellent for decongesting greasy, spotty and acneic skin.

Aromabeauty care
Bath p.m. • Facial care • Hair care • Hand care • Massage oil • Body compress • Vaporiser

ORANGE *(Citrus Aurantium)*
Family: *Rutaceae*

Plant: Tree
Part used: Peel of fruit
Extraction: Cold expression
Fragrance: Sweet and citrousy

Orange is a cheerful, uplifting oil that acts as a tonic to the nervous system. It is therefore a very useful oil in stress management. In beauty care, orange is a powerful disinfectant and cleanser, making it a very useful ingredient in an anti-cellulite blend for thighs and buttocks. Its eliminative powers make it ideal in the treatment of congested facial skin, and its benefits extend to the care of mature skin, as orange helps renew and regenerate cellular tissue.

Cautionary note: Orange is not to be used prior to sunbathing or using a sunbed as the skin may become more sensitive to burning and possible pigmentation.

Aromabeauty care:
Bath a.m. • Facial care • Hair care • Hand care • Massage oil • Vaporiser

PATCHOULI *(Pogostemon Patchouli)*
Family: *Labiatae*

Plant: Flowering shrub
Part used: Leaves
Extraction: Steam distillation
Fragrance: Earthy musky aroma

The perfume of the 'flower power' generation of the 1960s, patchouli is a thick oil with a persistant earthy aroma. Appealingly sensual, it has been known as an aphrodisiac since ancient times. In beauty care, patchouli has a marked effect on tissue regeneration, and is thus advocated for cases of acne and problem skins. Its healing powers and pleasing aroma make patchouli a perfect choice for fragrancing hand creams and for healing rough, damaged skin.

Aromabeauty Care
Bath p.m. • Facial care • Hair care • Hand care • Massage oil • Vaporiser

RAVANSARA *(Ravansara Aromatica)*
Family: *Lauraceae*

Plant: Medium-sized tree
Part used: Fruit and leaves
Extraction: Steam distillation
Fragrance: Cross between bay leaves and cloves

This little known oil, also called clove-nutmeg or Mada-
gascan nutmeg, is a remarkably effective anti-viral agent and
will inevitably become ever more popular in aromatherapy.
When resistance is low and the body needs a boost,
ravansara acts as a refreshing and strengthening tonic to
the whole system, making it particularly useful in the winter
months. In beauty care, its healing and sterilizing properties
make it a valuable addition to preparations for the treatment of acne and other skin problems.

Aromabeauty Care
Bath a.m. • Facial care • Massage oil • Body compress •
Vaporiser

ROSE *(Rosa Centifolia)*
Family: *Rosaceae*

Plant: Bush
Part used: Petals
Extraction: Solvent extraction yields absolute
Fragrance: Floral and characteristic

The flower of love, rose is healing on all levels – increasing
positive energy and overall feelings of well-being. This thick,
jewel-like red oil is the most sensual and inspiring of
fragrances. Rose imparts a profound sense of peace and
serenity, and is both relaxing and uplifting. In beauty care,
rose is a natural moisturizer and imbues the complexion
with a dewy softness. It is beneficial for all skin types. dry,
normal, mature and blemished. Because of its gentleness,
rose is especially suitable for sensitive skin. Rose is also
excellent for toning and firming body tissue due to its
astringent properties.

Aromabeauty Care
Bath p.m. • Facial care • Lip balm • Hand care • Massage
oil • Vaporiser

ROSEMARY *(Rosmarinus Officinalis)*
Family: *Labiateae*

Plant: Flowering shrub
Part used: Leaves and stems
Extraction: Steam distillation
Fragrance: Clear, camphoraceous

Perhaps the most stimulating of the essential oils, rosemary brings clarity when there is mental fatigue and restores energy to a tired body. It has been used since antiquity to strengthen and protect against negative influences, and as such plays a major role in combating stress today. In beauty care, rosemary helps tone tired muscles and revitalize dry, ageing skin. Its cleansing and antiseptic properties make it appropriate for treating acne and other skin blemishes. Rosemary is traditionally renowned as a hair tonic and restorer, especially so for dark hair.

Aromabeauty care
Bath a.m. • Facial care • Hair care • Massage oil • Vaporiser

SANDALWOOD *(Santalum Album)*
Family: *Santalaceae*

Plant: Tree
Part used: Heartwood
Extraction: Steam distillation
Fragrance: Warm and woody

This thick heavy oil with a long-lasting aroma has been used as incense in the East for thousands of years. A symbol of divine love and spirituality, as well as earthly love, sandalwood is a renowned aphrodisiac. On the emotional sphere, its effects are primarily sedative and calming, and it is thus commonly used to release stress and soothe anxiety. In beauty care, sandalwood oil is perfect for the treatment of combination skin. Its nourishing and moisturizing properties make it suitable for dry and mature skin, whilst its gentle astringent action helps with the treatment of oily and problem skin.

Aromabeauty care
Bath p.m • Facial care • Lip balm • Hair care • Hand care • Massage oil • Vaporiser

VETIVERT *(Andropogan Muricatus/Vetiveria Zizanoides)*
Family: *Gramineae*

Plant: Grass
Part used: Roots
Extraction. Steam distillation
Fragrance: Strong earthy aroma

Known as 'the oil of tranquility', vetivert imparts a sense of calm and peacefulness. It is therefore ideal in times of stress, tension and physical or mental exhaustion. With its deep lasting aroma, vetivert is not surprisingly a renowned aphrodisiac. In beauty care, the oil enables the skin to more readily retain water, making it one of nature's best moisturizers. Vetivert plumps out the tissues of the skin and helps to bring back a more youthful softness to mature skin.

Aromabeauty care
Bath p.m. • Facial care • Hand care • Massage oil

Ylang-ylang *(Cananga Odoratum)*
Family: *Anonaceae*

Plant: Tree
Part used: Flower
Extraction: Steam distillation
Fragrance: Exotic, floral

In the South Sea Islands where it is grown, ylang-ylang is called 'the flower of flowers'. The luxuriousness of its scent and its reputation for creating a mellow mood, combine to make ylang-ylang oil one of the world's most famous aphro-disiacs. The oil is excellent at counteracting negative emotions that cause stress, insomnia and nervous tension. In beauty care, ylang-ylang is a natural hair tonic, adding gloss and shine as well as a delightful perfume to the hair. On the skin, ylang-ylang is wonderfully balancing, enabling it to be used both for oily and dry skin.

Aromabeauty Care
Bath p.m. • Facial care • Hair care • Hand care • Massage oil • Vaporiser

Part B: Fatty oils

Essential oils must always be diluted in a fatty oil before use on the skin, and as there is a such a choice of fatty oils, it can be difficult to know which one to use.

Fatty oils contain essential fatty acids (EFAs), so called because they are needed by the body as part of our regular dietary intake. In this respect, we need to take in a variety of fatty acids, the most common ones being oleic acid, linoleic acid and linolenic acid. In beauty care, however, there is a different need. The need to choose a fatty oil which will not oxidize too readily is the primary concern, as oxidized fatty oils become home to free radicals which are dangerous to the cells of the body. When a massage oil (consisting of essential oils in a fatty oil base) becomes rancid, a chemical change takes place. This not only spoils the fragrance of the blend and prevents the essential oils from working properly, but if massaged into the skin, can introduce cell-damaging 'free radicals' into the body. It is also a waste of money.

Those fatty oils consisting primarily of oleic acid are called mono-unsaturated oils (mono meaning one) as this fatty acid only has one double bond in its chemistry. The higher the proportion of oleic acid, the more stable the oil. That is, it oxidizes much less slowly than fatty oils containing varying proportions of oleic and other fatty acids. When a fatty oil contains large amounts of the fatty acids linoleic and linolenic, the oil is known as a poly-unsaturated oil (poly meaning 'many') as these fatty acids have two and three double bonds respectively.

My first choice of fatty oil is camellia oil for several reasons – for its skin penetrating ability, its emollience, and its stability. And even though the cost is far greater than many other fatty oils, I cannot recommend it highly enough. My second choice is jojoba – technically not an oil but a liquid wax – also because of its fantastic keeping qualities as well as for its skin-beautifying and healing properties. My next choice is sweet almond oil.

Below is a chart of fatty oils, listing their oleic, linoleic and linolenic acid composition. Use the chart as a guide to buy the best oil that you can (i.e. the one nearest in composition to camellia), according to availability and the limitations of your budget.

CAMELLIA *(Camellia Japonica)*
Family: *Theaceae*

Plant: Evergreen tree
Part used: Seeds
Odour: Virtually odourless
Keeping qualities: Long lifespan. Very slow to oxidize as long as bottle is kept well-stoppered and out of sunlight.
Characteristics: A fairly thick but non-greasy oil with excellent skin-penetrating ability.

Camellia oil, as its full name suggests, comes from Japan, and is primarily cultivated on the islands of Izu and Kyushu. (*Camellia japonica* should not be confused with japonica or quince, which both belong to the *Rosaceae* family.) Its Japanese name is Tsubaki oil and is used in exclusive restaurants for cooking tempura – vegetables and prawns dipped in batter before quick frying – as the oil is very stable at high temperatures.

Camellia seeds, harvested in the autumn, are dried in the sun, crushed, roasted a little and then pressed to extract the oil. As this crude oil contains traces of water it is filtered and deodorised.

In beauty care the stability of camellia oil makes it by far the best fatty oil for facial and body use, as the dangers of rancidity and resultant 'free radicals' are negligible. It is instantly absorbed into the body and is non-greasy – leaving the skin feeling soft and emollient. The skin-penetrating properties of camellia oil enhance the speed at which diluted essential oils reach the deeper levels of the skin, and although expensive in terms of fatty oils, its cost is more than justified by its skin beautifying properties.

JOJOBA *(Simmondsia Chinensis/Californica)*
Family: *Simondsiaceae/Buxaceae*

Plant: Desert shrub
Part used: Nut
Odour: Pleasant nutty aroma
Keeping qualities: Excellent. Jojoba oil does not oxidize as it consists of 97 per cent wax esters with no glycerides and very little fatty acids.
Characteristics: Pale golden colour, with fairly thick consistency. The only plant in the world to contain a liquid wax.

For many years, jojoba has been favoured by North American Indians for its versatility – externally for the healing of sores and wounds, and internally for the relief of indigestion and constipation. Jojoba's anti-inflammatory effect is due to its myristic acid content, making it an effective treatment for rheumatism, arthritis and other swellings due to inflammation. French doctors practising aromatherapy administer essential oils by first diluting essences in jojoba oil and placing in capsules which are swallowed.

In beauty care, jojoba inhibits the production of excess sebum by imparting a light coating of wax to the skin, thus fooling the body into believing that enough sebum has been produced. It is this effect which makes jojoba a natural choice for treating acne and dandruff. Jojoba is also good for the treatment of dry hands, lips and facial skin as it contains nutrients which feed and regulate the skin's essential function. In hair care no other oil quite matches jojoba's ability to make hair look and feel healthy and lustrous. Jojoba oil gives some protection against the sun's rays as it has a sun-protection factor of 4.

ROSEHIP SEED *(Rosa Rubiginosa/Rosa Mosqueta)*
Family: *Rosaceae*

Plant: Rose bush from South America
Part used: Seeds of the rosehip
Odour: Strong, almost fish-oil aroma
Keeping qualities: 2 years unopened, 6 months when in use
Characteristics: Viscous oil with a golden-yellow colour

Rosehip seeds produce an oil which is rich in linoleic acid. This makes the oil vulnerable to oxidation and to counteract this effect, the oil is 'winterized' in order to reduce the number of fatty acids responsible for rancidity. Winterization is a process by which the oil is placed in cold temperatures to encourage the solidification of fatty acids which are then removed.

In beauty care, rosehip seed oil is valuable for use on mature skin, as it helps to prevent premature ageing. A little oil dotted around the outer eye area/cheekbone is an effective treatment for crow's feet. Rosehip seed oil is expensive in terms of fatty oils, and for this reason as well as because of its very strong aroma, only a small quantity of rosehip seed oil need be added to a facial massage oil. Dry skin as well as mature skin will benefit from the use of rosehip seed oil but because of its viscosity, it is not recommended for use on oily or acneic skins.

SWEET ALMOND *(Prunus Amygdalus)*
Family: *Rosaceae*

Plant: Tree
Part used: Nut
Odour: Almost odourless – bland
Keeping qualities: Fairly long-term if unopened as most sweet almond oil is refined to British Pharmacoepia standards. Once in use the oil will gradually break down as it oxidizes.
Characteristics: Very light golden colour and of medium sticky consistency.

Sweet almond oil is pressed from the kernels of the almond fruit and has been in use for thousands of years. First brought to Europe by the Romans, sweet almond oil has been used as an important ingredient in cosmetics ever since. It is a mono-unsaturated oil, containing approximately 70 per cent oleic acid which makes it less likely to oxidize and consequently one of the safest of the cheaper fatty oils.

In beauty care, sweet almond oil has softening and nourishing properties, and is a popular addition to face and hand creams. Because sweet almond oil is inexpensive, it is a good choice of oil in which to add more expensive fatty oils such as jojoba or rosehip seed. Sweet almond oil is an ideal oil for body massage, as its slightly sticky consistency gives the right amount of 'slip', and prevents immediate absorption by the skin.

Fatty Oils Chart					
Oil		% Oleic	% Linoleic	% Linolenic	
Almond (sweet)	M	70	20	—	N
Apricot	M/P	65	27	—	N
Avocado	M	70	9	—	N
Camellia	M	78-92	1-2.2	—	N
Coconut	Sat	6.5	1.5	—	—
Corn	P	19-49	34-62	0-2.7	S
Cotton seed	P	15.3-36	35-54.8	—	S
Grapeseed	P	14	74	—	S
Hazelnut	M	77	10	—	N
Olive	M	65-85	3.9-15	0-1	N
Peach kernel	M/P	68	25	—	N
Peanut	M	42.3-61.1	13-33.4	—	N
Pumpkin	P	35	45	—	S
Rapeseed *	P	12-18	12-16	7-9	S
Rice	P	40-50	29-42	0-1	S
Rosehip seed	P	15	47	28-30	N
Safflower	P	13	75	—	S
Sesame	M	35-46	35.2-48.4	0.2	N
Soyabean	P	23.5-30.8	49.2-52	1.9-10	D
Sunflower	P	33	52	0-1	S
Walnut	P	15	55	10-12	S
Jojoba – liquid wax					

Key

M   mono-unsaturated   Sat saturated
P   poly-unsaturated   N   non-drying
M/P borderline between mono-unsaturated   S   semi-drying
      and poly-unsaturated   D   drying
* N.B. Rapeseed oil should not be used at all.

Glossary

Adrenaline Hormone produced by adrenal glands in response to stress or fear. It raises the blood pressure and utilizes sugars to provide instant energy.

Adrenals Adrenal glands, located on top of the kidneys, manufacture over 40 hormones.

Anabolism The building up of new body requirements – muscle or energy – from simple compounds. Anabolic steroids are produced by the adrenals. This stimulates metabolism to form sugars and proteins which in turn create new cell growth.

Catabolism Metabolic change of nutrients which causes a breaking down of complex substances into simpler compounds, which can be used by the body as fuel for energy.

Cellulite Term used to describe the 'orange peel' effect found most commonly on women's thighs. Caused by an excess of toxins in the body, these toxins invade tissue cells making them permeable. Not to be confused with **Cellulitis** which is a skin infection (literally an inflamation of cells of the skin) due to presence of germs.

Collagen Organic constitutent of bone, cartilage and connective tissue. Animal collagen is often added to commercial beauty creams.

Dehydration Loss of water content.

Distillation Method of extracting essential oils from plants by the use of pressurized steam.

EFAs Essential fatty acids. Components of all fatty oils.

Effleurage Gentle sweeping massage strokes, used after application of aromatic oil to the body. Soft tissue massage of the body or face.

Emollient Skin softening oil.

Expression Extracting essential oils from citrus peel by pressing.

Free radical Destructive oxygen particle which causes degeneration of tissues, i.e. a chemical change takes place when fatty oil is oxygenated (it becomes rancid).

Gland An organ that forms and releases (secretes) substances that act elsewhere; endocrine or exocrine. A gland is an endocrine if the secretion is internal, i.e. hormones from the adrenal glands. Exocrine glands secrete to the outside, i.e. sweat glands release sweat to the skin.

Hydrophobic Something which has an aversion to water, such as essential oils.

Linoleic acid One of the essential fatty acids. Known as one of the poly-unsaturated fatty acids as it contains more than one double bond. The human body can convert linoleic acid into gamma-linoleic acid (GLA).

Linolenic acid One of the EFAs known as a poly-unsaturated fatty acid. A colourless liquid glycerine found in most oils.

Lipophilic Something which has an affinity to oils and fats, such as essential oils.

Lymph Colourless fluid with many of the characteristics of blood, and which forms part of the circulatory system. Lymph permeates body tissues, draining off bacteria and other toxins, and bringing protective lymphocytes. It travels through lymph capillaries, lymph conducting vessels and lymph transport vessels. Similar to veins, the transport vessels contain valvular segments which force the lymph along the main trunks and thoracic duct and return it to the bloodstream at the angle of the clavicle and base of the neck.

Lymph node Another name for lymph gland. Small bean-shaped glands that produce lymphocytes and act as filters to help remove unwanted toxins etc from the body. At any one time, only 2 per cent of all lymphocytes are travelling through the bloodstream, whilst 98 per cent are bathing the interstitial connective tissues.

Meridians Another name for 'channels of energy' referred to in Chinese medicine (acupressure, acupuncture) and Japanese shiatsu.

Metabolism The chemical change that converts food into compounds which can be used by the body to rebuild and replenish cells, as fuel for energy, and to break down waste products into substances that can be eliminated. Metabolism constists of catabolism and anabolism.

Mono-unsaturated fat See 'oleic acid'.

Obesity Excessive weight being detrimental to health. Cause is usually a combination of poor metabolism and consumption of too much fat-rich foods which accumulate in the body.

Oedema An excessive collection of fluid within the body tissues. Can be caused by sluggish circulation, too much salt in the diet or lymphatic system not functioning correctly.

Oleic acid One of the essential fatty acids. Called a mono-unsaturated fatty acid because it contains only one double bond.

Photosensitization An essential oil which, when applied to the skin, makes the skin more sensitive to the sun's rays and therefore can be damaged more easily.

Poly-unsaturated fats See linoleic acid and linolenic acid.

Rubefacient An essential oil which when applied to the skin (even in dilution) causes local heat.

Shiatsu Ancient Japanese system of healing that unblocks and balances the flow of energy to the body's vital organs by applying pressure to certain channels of energy and specific points along those channels.

Select Bibliography

Old Age: its cause and prevention. The story of an old body and face made young Sanford Bennett
The Physical Culture Publishing Co, New York, 1912

The Fat Factor John O'Mullane and Carol Muir
Thorsons, 1986

Jojoba and Yucca Frena Bloomfield
Century Hutchinson, 1985

A Consumers Dictionary of Cosmetic Ingredients Ruth Winter
Crown Publishers Inc, New York, 1989

Let's Get Well Adelle Davis
George Allen and Unwin Ltd, London, 1974

The Book of Shiatsu Paul Lundberg
Gaia Books Ltd, 1992

Aromatherapy for Women Maggie Tisserand
Thorsons (HarperCollins), 1985, 1990, 1993

Slim Well (with the new cellulite cure) Joan Clayton
Kenneth Mason, 1979

A Natural History of the Senses Diane Ackerman
Chapmans, 1990

Books by the same author

Aromatherapy for Women
Thorsons (HarperCollins), 1985, 1990, 1993

The Magic and Power of Lavender
Schneelowe Verlag, Munich, 1989

Aromatherapy for Lovers
Thorsons (HarperCollins), 1993

Useful Addresses

Camellia, jojoba and rosehip seed oils, plus a large selection of essential oils, green clay, etc., may be obtained by post from:

Maggie Tisserand
8 Paston Place
Brighton BN2 1HA

tel: 0273 693622
fax: 0273 676677

Vitamin E oil may be obtained by post from:

House of Mistry
15-17 South End Road
Hampstead Heath
London NW3 2PT

tel: 071 794 0848

Kaolin and fuller's earth are available from most chemists. Beeswax is available from many hardware stores.
Sweet almond oil can be found in many health food stores and chemists.

Index

Acknowledgements

My grateful thanks go to the following people:

Elizabeth Millar for her help and support with the writing of this book.

Dr. Peter Helps M.B., B.S., Dip. Ac., M.R.T.C.M. for his medical expertise.

Paul Lundberg B.Ac., M.R.T.C.M., M.R.S.S. for his shiatsu advise.

Lucy and Saffron, my teenage daughters, for their help with the planning of the teenage skin section. Special thanks to Lucy for her enthusiasm and help with formulating and making hand creams in our kitchen.

Jan Kusmerik of Natural Active Materials Research Ltd (N.A.M.R.) for his help in compiling the fatty acids chart.